Grow Young with Your Dog

Learn How You and Your Canine
Companion Can Feel Better at Any Age!

Mary Debono, GCFP
Creator of *Debono Moves*^{sm}

DebonoMoves.com

Ruby Red Press

Published by Ruby Red Press

Printed in the United States of America
Published November 2014

Second Printing: 2015

Disclaimers

The information in this book is true and complete to the best of our knowledge. This book is intended only as an informative guide for those wishing to learn more about canine and human health and mobility. In no way is this book intended to replace, countermand or conflict with the advice given to you by your own physician or your dog's veterinarian. Decisions concerning care for you and your dog should be made between you and your health professionals. We strongly recommend that you follow medical advice.

Dogs are unpredictable and may be dangerous. *Do not proceed in touching any dog who may be unsafe.*

Information in this book is general and is offered with no guarantees on the part of the author, SENSE Method, Inc., or Ruby Red Press.

The author and publisher disclaim all liability in connection with the use of this book. Consult with a qualified health professional before starting a movement program for you or your dog.

For my beloved parents,
Edgar and Teresa Debono

Grow Young with Your Dog

Praise for Mary Debono

"Mary combines an amazing knowledge of anatomy, movement, structure, behavior combined with love, empathy and observation. Best of all she is articulate and a good communicator. This book will forever change how you view not only your dog, but all animals! It will forever change how you interact with your dog and all animals, including humans!! **– Tina Steward, D.V.M.**

"This is a wonderful book for every dog owner, not just for their dog but for themselves too. I've been lucky enough to study with Mary and experienced firsthand her excellent and caring teaching. I use her teachings with the dogs and horses who are my clients. The exercises are straightforward, well explained and mindful. Your dog will appreciate you using your hands in the gentle ways that Mary describes. Do the exercises for yourself and gain an understanding of why animals and humans love Mary's work." **– Elizabeth Sleight**

"I have had the pleasure of working with Mary for several years, and I can't recommend her work enough. I can personally attest to the wonderful changes I have seen in dogs (and horses) using her work. I'm so happy more people will be introduced to Mary and her work through this book!" **– Leah Astrup**

"Excellent information that heals the dog and enriches the person in many ways. This approach is another valuable tool in the alternative healing toolbox. I've known Mary Debono and her work for some time. Clearly written, informative and pleasantly illustrated. Mary lifts the veil and shows us what she does and how she does in an easy to follow manner. An opportunity to learn the anatomy of a dog and by extension our own." **– Brigitte Noel, Author of LoveLink: Heart to Heart Communication with Animals**

"I know I've said it before, and I'm sure I'll say it again – you are incredible. What you are able to do is amazing. My dog Misty is feeling so much better and she wants to play again. It's so wonderful to see how much better she feels. Thank you again." **– Cathy Dameron**

"My 13-year-old dog Roscoe was having lots of stiffness and pain from arthritis. Roscoe absolutely loves his Debono Moves sessions and I have noticed so much improvement in his walking. He has stopped favoring his right front leg and he really wants to go for short walks once again." – **Leslie Johnson Leech**

"I am thrilled and amazed at how quickly my mind and body has integrated the movements and that I am now almost totally pain free. Unbelievable that it went that fast. I have had whole body pain for about 5 years." – **Rosemary Melsey**

"Mary Debono brings such integrity, passion, and skill to her work with animals and people. She has an exquisite understanding of energy and movement. I have thoroughly enjoyed working with such a skilled teacher and healer." – **Sharon B. Franklin, D.V.M.**

"I cannot thank you enough for all that you offered me and my dog, Charlie Brown. I truly believe that your touch helped Charlie Brown be much, much more comfortable, relaxed, and restful. After your sessions, he walked better and was noticeably more comfortable in his own body. Thank you!!!" – **Julie Lively**

"I am a disabled veteran with PTSD. My service dog gets overwhelmed with my symptoms. I feel sometimes I take and ask so much of him, he gets burned out. I watched your video and now he is following me everywhere. I did Debono Moves on his neck in the sit position and he went to sleep in my hands, still sitting up. You are onto something big, if people would slow down and listen to their animals." – **Tim Taylor**

"What you taught us in your workshop about the listening touch has been quite helpful with my dog. I was sitting on the bed with her draped over my lap, and I wanted to work on her. I put my hand on her ribs, and she immediately went into a panicky "something bad is going to happen" mode. So I just left my hand there without doing anything else, and after a few minutes, she got comfortable enough to let me do more. I could see she was starting to enjoy herself, and at one point, she let out a big sigh and seemed deeply relaxed; she eventually fell asleep. I've been able to do the same thing with other procedures that make her uncomfortable." – **A.T.**

"Mary, I wanted to let you know that Tony is so much better this morning. He's using his right front leg properly and not dragging his toe so much. You work miracles. Thanks!" **– Janie Emerson**

"Sensitive, intelligent work that will surely help your dog." **– Jan Rasmusen, Author**

"This work makes you appreciate how small changes bring about big improvements in comfort and movement. You don't need to build muscle or stretch for improvement to occur." **– Dr. Shirley Strum, noted anthropologist**

To read more endorsements of Mary's work, please visit http://www.debonomoves.com/testimonials.

Grow Young with Your Dog

Acknowledgements

This book has been percolating for a long time. I was just a young child when I began to wonder how I could improve the well-being of animals and their human companions. I knew it involved using my hands. But I didn't know *how*.

Several years later I began to intuitively explore using my hands to help animals feel better and move more freely. The astonishing part was that it benefited *me* as much as the animals I was trying to help! I knew then that I was onto something.

Along the way, I studied various ways to promote health and well-being. Some of them resonated strongly with me and I translated their concepts to animals. One such approach was the *Feldenkrais Method®*, www.Feldenkrais.com, of somatic education. I am forever grateful to the late Dr. Moshe Feldenkrais for developing his groundbreaking work and for passing it down to his students, who became my teachers. Thank you all. I especially thank Lawrence Phillips, www.OneBodySpirit.net, who as my first *Feldenkrais* teacher helped me realize how much change is truly possible.

I am thankful for the many animals who put themselves in my hands. I have learned so much from each and every one. I extend gratitude to all the people who trusted me with their beloved dogs, cats, rabbits and horses. I thank the students who came from near and far to attend my workshops so that they could discover how to help their own animals. Their enthusiasm and zest for learning helped shape *Debono Moves*.

I thank you, dear reader, for picking up this book and embarking upon a journey to wellness with your dog. I hope we meet – even virtually – sometime soon. It's exciting that technology is allowing the *Debono Moves* community to connect with each other, no matter where we live.

I also wish to thank:

Betsy Seeton, www.LiveHonestly.com, for her editorial expertise and helpful suggestions;

Mary VanMeer, VirtualAssistantGazette.com, who cheerfully and skillfully formatted the book and expertly updated my website;

Kathy Upton, www.AgilityVideos4You.com, a talented graphic designer, photographer and canine agility competitor, who took many of the photos that appear throughout this book; and

Vicki Armstrong, dog rescuer and flyball maven, www.coastalexpressflyball.com, for her enthusiastic support, friendship and for lending her beautiful dogs for a photo shoot.

I thank my parents for modeling love and care for all living beings, and for giving me the indelible joy of growing up with our much-loved family dog. I thank my dad for all the time we spent going to dog shows and obedience trials. I am grateful to my sisters, friends and extended family for their continued love and support. I thank the animals who have shared my heart and home, filling my soul with love and laughter.

And, last but certainly not least, I thank my beloved husband, Gary Waskowsky, www.GaryWaskowsky.com, for all his love, support, boundless wisdom, photography, videography and dog walking. This book would not be possible without you, Sweetie.

Table of Contents

Praise for Mary Debono iii

Acknowledgements vii

Introduction 1

An Important Note to the Reader 5

Chapter One: A Canine Mission Impossible? 7

  A Poodle On a Mission...7

  Guidelines for Doing the Exercises 12

    Find a Comfortable, Quiet Spot to Do the Exercises....12

    There Is No "Correct" Way to Do the Movements.......13

    Take a Break Before Moving on to the Next Exercise .13

    Move with Mindfulness All Day 13

    Let Comfort Be Your Guide 14

    Small, Slow Movements Equal Big Improvements......14

    Breathe Easily 14

    Rest Frequently 15

    Embrace Novelty 15

    Use Your Imagination...15

  Are You Really Comfortable? 16

  Key Points of Chapter One 16

Chapter Two: A Healing Connection Helps an Older Dog Walk Again...19

  Rocky Improves – And So Do I 19

  Connected Breathing 24

The Healing Power of Connection 30

Human Exercise #1: Deeper Breath, Lighter Hands 31

Getting to Know Your Dog in a New Way 32

    The Front Leg 33

    The Shoulder Blade 33

    The Ribs 35

    The Sternum 35

    The Spine 37

    The Hind Leg 37

    The Hip Joint 38

    The Ischium 39

    The Head 40

Human Exercise #2: Improve Your Walking by Lying Down 41

Key Points of Chapter Two 41

Chapter Three: Improved Back Flexibility Got These Dogs Moving Again 43

    Cassie Overcomes Spinal Arthritis 43

    Mary Writes About Cassie 46

Recovering from a Chronic Muscle Injury 49

Human Exercise #3: Easier Sitting 51

Make It All About You and Your Dog 52

Back Lifts 53

Ribcage Rolls 58

Human Exercise #4: Lengthen Your Hamstrings Without Stretching 60

Key Points of Chapter 3 61

Chapter Four: Getting Rid of a Pain in the Neck 63

A Neck Injury Doesn't Stop this Canine Athlete 63

Learning for Life...69

Human Exercise #5: Stirring the Soup 70

Ribcage Circles..71

Shoulder and Ribcage Circles..77

Human Exercise #6: Turning Toward a Supple Spine 80

Key Points of Chapter Four...81

Chapter Five: What Do Torn Knee Ligaments, Arthritis, and Habits Have in Common? 83

Sonny Heals His Torn Knee Ligament................................83

Jackson Stops Arthritis in Its Tracks 89

Scanning Your Dog's Body..94

Standing 95

Sitting...96

Lying Down 96

Human Exercise #7: Hip and Shoulder Circles 97

Hip and Shoulder Circles...97

When Good Habits Go Bad 101

Taking Off Your Pants Can Keep You Nimble...............102

Think Yourself Younger...107

Key Points of Chapter Five..110

Chapter Six: From Hip Dysplasia to Agility 113

A Young Dog Overcomes Hip Dysplasia.........................113

Managing Hip Dysplasia in the Active Dog....................121

How to Help an Anxious or Distracted Dog 122

Human Exercise #8: Making Time for Freer Hips......... 127

Human Exercise #9: Sitting on a Clock 127

Muscle Lifts.. 127

Shoulder Blade 130

Lower Leg 131

Hindquarters 132

Muscle Rolls... 133

Key Points of Chapter Six 137

Chapter Seven: Enhancing the Life of the Older Dog 139

Geriatric Dog Learns How to Wag Her Tail Again 139

Hope for an Older Dog Who Could No Longer Stand.... 141

Lumbar Lifts... 148

Lumbar Circles... 150

Add More Time to Your Life ... And More Life to Your Time 152

The Seven Suggestions.. 153

Exercise #10: Better Posture Effortlessly..................... 155

Key Points of Chapter Seven 155

Chapter Eight: Human Exercises 157

Human Exercise #1: Deeper Breath, Lighter Hands 157

Human Exercise #2: Improve Your Walking by Lying Down 162

Human Exercise #3: Easier Sitting................................ 170

Variations 177

Human Exercise #4: Lengthen Your Hamstrings Without Stretching 177

Variation 182

Human Exercise #5: Stirring the Soup 184

Variation 188

Human Exercise #6: Turning Toward a Supple Spine ...189

Human Exercise #7: Hip and Shoulder Circles 196

Variations...206

Human Exercise #8: Making Time for Freer Hips 207

Human Exercise #9: Sitting on a Clock......................211

Variations...216

Human Exercise #10: Better Posture Effortlessly 216

Resources...227

Educational Products and Classes 227

Free Newsletter 227

Workshops and Clinics 227

Private Sessions 227

Find a *Feldenkrais Method*® Practitioner 228

Locate a Holistic Veterinarian 228

Dog Training..228

Meet the Dogs! 229

About the Author...231

Grow Young with Your Dog

Introduction

Do you feel older today than you did 25 years ago? Many people respond to that question with, *"Of course I feel older!"* They *expect* to feel older with the passage of time, and they have the stiffness, pains, and limitations to prove it.

What makes *you* feel older? Are you no longer able to do activities that you once enjoyed, such as hiking up a mountain, running through a forest or kayaking through white water? Or is it difficult to do even mundane things like taking a long walk, going up and down stairs or sitting on the floor? Is your balance not as good as it once was? Do you generally get stiff and achy and assume that's what "getting older" feels like?

Is your state of mind "old"? Do you tend to worry and obsess over things? Do you feel stuck in some part of your life? When was the last time you acted spontaneously? Have you lost your curiosity and optimism about life?

When I was in my late 20's I suffered from a variety of aches and pains. I had bi-lateral carpal tunnel syndrome that resulted in nerve damage, a very painful hip, and stiffness in my back and neck. As I was rubbing my sore lower back one day, I thought, "Well, I have to expect this. I'm getting older." For goodness' sake, I was in my twenties! Although quite a number of years have passed since that day, I feel younger *now* than I did back then.

Over the past 25+ years I've learned a lot about how to feel and move more youthfully.[1] I learned that when we stay stuck in our habitual ways of thinking and moving we get *physically* stuck too. We develop sore muscles and stiff joints. We hesitate to explore new activities. We lose our balance and

---

[1] My studies have included biomechanics, anatomy, energetic medicine, behavioral science and the *Feldenkrais Method®* of Somatic Education. While they all aided in forming *Debono Moves^sm*, the greatest contribution comes from Dr. Moshe Feldenkrais' teachings.

become afraid to fall. We fuss and worry about some version of the same old thing decade after decade. We become limited in our thoughts and limited in our movements. In short, we feel *old*.

To grow younger, I released the habits that kept me stuck in unhealthy patterns, and I learned to think and act in different ways. I discovered that it's the *newness* of our thoughts, sensations and movements that help the brain continue to grow and develop as we age. Both in mind and body, *novelty* is the key to expanding our abilities. And that helps us feel *young*.

As dog lovers, we want the same thing for our dogs. We'd like our dogs to be happy, healthy and active for as long as possible. *In short, we want our dogs to grow young with us.* After all, what fun would a hike up a mountain be without your beloved canine romping by your side?

That's why I developed *Debono Moves*[sm] and wrote this book to share it.[2] *Debono Moves* is an approach that you can easily use to help yourself and your dog feel better and move more joyfully. In this book I describe how I have helped dogs heal completely from injuries and surgeries, move well despite arthritis and hip dysplasia, recover from a paralyzing stroke and run and play again after being classified as "too old to recover."

Debono Moves combines the science of neuroplasticity, the ability of the brain to overcome injury or disease by forming new neural pathways, with the healing power of love. This potent synergy helps us achieve higher levels of functioning, connection and awareness with our animal companions.

Using gentle contact and supportive movements, you will learn how to:

- Reduce stress and anxiety
- Minimize the risk of injury

---

[2] *Debono Moves*[sm] was formerly known as the *SENSE Method*.

- Comfort the aging and infirm
- Improve athletic performance
- Enhance vitality and well-being
- Facilitate healing after injury, surgery or illness
- Cultivate a deep bond between human and canine
- Lessen the effects of arthritis, hip dysplasia and aging

One of the unique characteristics of *Debono Moves* is that it is designed to help you improve right along with your dog. That's why this book is accompanied by easy-to-do exercises that can help rid you of stiffness, stress, aches and poor posture, while gaining flexibility, better balance and improved coordination. In short, you'll feel *younger*.

I think of this program as investing in yourself and your dog, because what you do *today* will affect how you'll feel in ten or more years. Taking the time to move more comfortably *now* can reduce wear and tear on joints and muscles in the future. In a nutshell, *it's never too early to start feeling younger*.

But it's also *never too late* to start! Several of the dogs portrayed in this book were at an advanced age with a poor prognosis when I met them. But yet they improved their abilities considerably. These plucky dogs taught me that regardless of age or physical condition, you can improve your quality of life. This is true for humans and canines alike.

With this book in hand, you no longer have to choose between spending quality time with your dog and taking care of yourself. As you do the basic techniques with your dog, you may discover that your body moves more freely, your mind is calmer and clearer, and your spirit more joyful.

Wouldn't you like to grow young with your dog? Well, let's get started!

Grow Young with Your Dog

An Important Note to the Reader

You're probably familiar with approaches such as massage and chiropractic which aim to change the muscles or skeleton. *Debono Moves*, which I introduce in this book, is quite different. In *Debono Moves*, hands are used not to manipulate, but to *communicate*. This is a big distinction. The intent for this gentle, tactile communication is to *awaken new possibilities for canine movement and behavior*. The dogs themselves actually create the change.

Using this book, you can learn twelve basic *Debono Moves* to do with your dog. And while there are many dogs who have experienced the benefits of these moves, your results may differ. Outcomes can be affected by your dog's particular situation and your expertise in doing the moves. As you explore the lessons in this book, please move slowly and gently, and always ensure that you and your dog are comfortable.

To illustrate the remarkable possibilities for canine improvement, I tell the stories of dogs who have overcome the effects of injury, stroke, hip dysplasia, arthritis and aging.[3] I am not implying that these results are typical or that you'll duplicate them. And while I detail the hands-on strategies I used to help these dogs, it is beyond the scope of this book to teach the advanced techniques that I employed. So unless you have additional training in *Debono Moves,* please do not attempt to imitate the sessions I describe.

If you would like increase your ability to help your dog, please visit www.DebonoMoves.com for information on educational workshops, products and our free newsletter[4].

---

[3] To meet these dogs online, visit www.DebonoMoves.com/Products/Dog-Book.

[4] Our newsletter provides *free* articles and videos to help you and your dogs, cats and horses.

Debono Moves is a *system of improvement* designed to enhance body awareness, comfort and movement, while deepening the human-canine bond. It is not a substitute for medical treatment. The canines portrayed in this book were under the care of veterinarians, and the stories and suggestions are for educational purposes only. Consult with a qualified health professional if either you or your dog is ill or injured.

Debono Moves is a fun, satisfying way to feel better at any age, and I'm excited to share it with you. Thank you for embarking on this journey to wellness with your dog!

Chapter One: A Canine Mission Impossible?

It's 6 a.m. and your dog is whining to go out. You roll your tired, achy body out of bed, grimacing as your feet hit the floor. The first steps are always so stiff. Your dog is circling now, barking at you to hurry up. *"All right, all right! I'm coming as fast as I can!"* you bark back. At times like this, you think, *"Ugh! Getting older stinks."*

Many people have told me a version of this story. They assume that they are too old, too arthritic or too injured to ever feel any better. And they assume the same is true about their dogs. They have been led to believe that certain conditions only get worse. Never better. But I don't deal with "conditions." I work with animals and their humans. And with the right help, many of them *can* feel better, even against some pretty steep odds. Here's the story of one of them. Buttons was a little white dog who taught me that even an old, infirm dog can improve. Perhaps she'll inspire you to think differently about what is possible for you and your dog.

A Poodle On a Mission

Making the impossible possible. Apparently that was my assignment on a rainy Sunday evening. I had just gotten a phone call about a poodle that had suffered a stroke ten days before while undergoing surgery. The caller, Clare, was close to tears as she told me that her veterinarian held no hope for the dog's recovery, and was strongly recommending euthanasia. But Clare and her husband wanted to make sure that they gave their girl every chance, so when a friend told them about my work, Clare immediately picked up her phone and anxiously asked if I could come over that night.[5]

As soon as I got off the phone with Clare, I checked my map, got into my red Celica and headed to La Jolla. It was wintertime and the evening rain had gone from a drizzle to a downpour. As I merged onto I-5, the wipers moved rhythmically across the windshield and I thought about how I might help this elderly poodle. What could I do that veterinary medicine could not? Would I be able to enhance the quality of life of this little dog? I remembered the desperation in Clare's voice and felt a great weight of responsibility.

After I exited the freeway and turned onto the rain-slicked streets of the upscale beach town, I heard waves crashing against the shore. Even though a light rain was still falling, I opened the windows to let in the ocean breeze. I breathed deeply, relishing the smell of the sea. Ever since moving to California, I associated the ocean with optimism and rebirth. Having spent many years working in windowless offices on the East Coast, I was still somewhat amazed that I was actually living in Southern California. I had left a lucrative, but unfulfilling, career in computer systems to pursue my life's passion – helping animals and their people. And here I was, living my dream. The Pacific Ocean was a reminder of how far I had come and why I was here. My life was proof that transformation is possible, as long as you open your heart and mind to the possibility. This recollection restored my sense of tranquility as I looked for Clare's house.

I found the large, oceanfront house and parked in the circular driveway. I had hardly begun to knock when the door was opened by a 50-something-year-old woman with short, dark hair. Clare had the tanned, fit look of someone who enjoyed walking on the beach. But her sad eyes and trembling lips conveyed the ache in her heart. Clare invited me in and

---

[5] This story, like the others in this book, is true. However, the names in this chapter have been changed as I was unable to contact the individuals involved to obtain permission to publish their names.

introduced me to her husband Frank, a grey-haired man wearing a maroon polo shirt and khakis. Frank's brow was furrowed with worry as he shook my hand.

I entered the spacious living room and looked around for the dog. My breath caught in my throat when I saw her. The white miniature poodle was lying on a pink quilt laid over clear plastic sheeting. Her eyes were closed and she didn't move a muscle when I entered the room. In fact, I had to look very closely to see if the skinny little dog was even breathing. Buttons was in much worse shape than I had expected.

Clare, red-eyed and morose, filled me in on the details. Buttons, 15 years old, had barely moved since awakening from general anesthesia ten days ago. Although the surgery to remove her spleen had been uneventful, when Buttons awoke she could no longer bear weight on her left legs. They remained stick-straight, unable to bend. Her neck and back were severely restricted in movement and radiographs revealed extensive deterioration of the vertebrae.

As Clare and Frank took a seat on the large sofa, I made myself comfortable on the floor next to Buttons. Frank told me that I was their dog's last hope. If I couldn't help her, they had agreed to put her to sleep. I explained that I didn't know how much I could help their beloved little girl, but I would do what I could. To buy some time, I agreed to work with Buttons only if they committed to three sessions, spaced out every other day. After that we could evaluate the dog's progress. They readily agreed to my plan.

This occurred in January of 1995, almost two decades ago. Although I had been working professionally with animals for several years by then, I had never worked with a dog that had suffered a stroke. In fact, as Clare and Frank waited for me to produce a miracle, I wasn't at all sure of what I was going to do. I knew that I could help the poodle feel at least a little bit better, but beyond that, I hadn't a clue.

Taking a deep breath, I took stock of what I *did* know. I knew that gentle, rhythmic movements seem to help "reset" a traumatized nervous system. I had once been on the receiving end of such movements and was amazed at how they helped me recover after an accident[6]. Ever since, I have been using them successfully with animals; so that night, with Buttons, rebooting her system is where I began.

Using my fingertips, I made a gentle, rhythmic exploration of the little dog's entire body. I felt how easy it was to delicately flex Buttons' right legs, but her left legs were stiff and unbending, as if she was in rigor mortis. The poodle had been unable to control her left side since her stroke.

I worked very gently, checking for the subtlest sign that Buttons was responding to my touch. In a short while, I noticed that her breathing became deeper. We were connecting! I hoped that she was developing more awareness of her body and awakening areas that had been "turned off." When I left Buttons that night, she was resting peacefully.

Clare greeted me enthusiastically on Tuesday, saying that Buttons had gotten up on her own after Sunday's session. This intelligent little dog had begun to use their large circular sofa as a crutch, allowing it to support her left side as her functioning right legs slowly motored her around.

Buttons' responses at our second session were clearer and I knew we were making progress. How much she would improve, however, was still an unknown. As I brought the session to a close, the white dog rose to her feet. Leaning against the sofa, Buttons slowly walked around. Gradually she moved away from the sofa's support and took three steps. Although she remained stiff-legged and weak, it was quite an accomplishment.

It was a sunny, blustery day when I visited Buttons for the third time. I felt the little dog's left legs, which were still rigid and unyielding. Then I worked with her right legs, which bent

---

[6] I experienced the profound healing effect of gentle, intentional, rhythmic movements during a *Feldenkrais® Functional Integration®* session with Sharon Starika in the early 1990's.

easily at the joints. I crossed the poodle's front legs, so that her left front leg was on the right side of her body and her right front leg was on the left side. And then I *imagined* that her left legs were her right legs, and vice versa.

As I held this image, I touched the joints of her left front leg, testing if they would bend. And, lo and behold, they did! Bending the left foreleg had been *impossible* until I moved it across her midline. I crossed her hind legs too, and had the same, fascinating result[7]!

As I was bringing Thursday's session to a close, Buttons got up. This time the poodle didn't use the sofa as a crutch. She simply stood up on her own. I noticed immediately that her left legs had lost their rigidity and had healthy joint angles. But I gasped as I caught sight of her right legs, which were held as rigid as steel rods. Before I could put my hands on her, the poodle relaxed her right legs and began walking across the carpet, as if it was the most natural thing in the world. Whew!

It was at this moment that Clare entered the room and saw her dog walking unaided. Teary-eyed, she began shouting, "*I wish we had before and after videos!*" Well, yes, me too! It was quite a dramatic moment.

While it would be amazing enough that this dog recovered her ability to walk, what really rocked my world was that for at least one heart-stopping moment, her **right** side became the stiff, unmoving side. This clearly demonstrated just how plastic, or malleable, the nervous system is. *And since the nervous system controls all of our functioning, this makes our potential for improvement very great indeed.*

---

[7] I learned about the usefulness of taking limbs across the midline from the work of Dr. Moshe Feldenkrais, the originator of the *Feldenkrais Method®*. Dr. Feldenkrais, who worked solely with humans, had great success with helping people recover their functioning after stroke and other trauma. Crossing the limbs may stimulate the nervous system to form new neural connections, and I have since used this strategy with other dogs suffering from paralysis due to stroke.

Buttons never needed another *Debono Moves* session. I checked on her a couple of months later and she was still walking around her house and yard just fine. Although it's been almost two decades since she took those dramatic steps, I'll never forget the little white poodle who was one of my greatest teachers. *This fifteen-year-old dog demonstrated that learning and improving are possible regardless of advanced age or weakened physical condition.* And while I was honored to be a partner in her recovery, it was the dog, not I, who transformed *impossible* into *possible.* Mission accomplished, Buttons!

Guidelines for Doing the Exercises

Like Buttons, you can improve your movement too. To experience how easily your brain can be rewired for more youthful movement, please explore the non-traditional exercises that accompany this book, which are inspired by *Feldenkrais Method*® *Awareness Through Movement*® lessons.

The exercises appear in printed form, accompanied by photos, in the last section of this book. For your convenience in following the instructions, I also provide audio recordings of the exercises.

Before you dive in, please note the following recommend-dations which apply to *all* the exercises.

Find a Comfortable, Quiet Spot to Do the Exercises

You will benefit more if you are not distracted while doing each awareness exercise. Find a time and a place where you won't be disturbed. Close the door and turn off your cell phone. Wear comfortable clothes, such as yoga or sweat pants. Take off your shoes and remove any jewelry, eyeglasses, belts, watches and the like.

If it is a sitting exercise, make sure you have a firm, flat-bottomed chair to use. If you will be lying down, make sure the floor is carpeted or that you have a comfortable blanket or soft mat handy. Have a couple of folded towels nearby to place it behind your head when you are lying down. Adjust the temperature of the room before you start.

There Is No "Correct" Way to Do the Movements

Use the photos as a guide, but do not try to imitate the movement exactly as it is shown. The exercises are designed to help you feel *how you move*, so that you can release inefficient habits and make your movements lighter and easier.

Take a Break Before Moving on to the Next Exercise

Relax, take a walk or do some other quiet activity before moving on to the next exercise. This gives your brain time to integrate the movements. Mindfully doing one or two of the exercises a day will be more beneficial than doing several hurriedly. Take your time and don't rush through them.

Move with Mindfulness All Day

These awareness exercises can help develop your ability to be more attentive to yourself. You'll progress faster if you bring this observant nature to your everyday life too. When you are in front of your computer or driving your car, notice how you are sitting. When you are walking your dog, notice how your arms swing, how your feet hit the ground and how you are holding your dog's leash. Discover where you can release unnecessary tension, including your shoulders, facial muscles, fingers and toes.

Explore how you can make all of your positions and movements easier and more comfortable throughout the day. Notice how the exercises that accompany this book improve your ability to stand, walk, reach, sit and breathe.

Let Comfort Be Your Guide

Move only as much as is easy and comfortable for you. Pain can create tension and other unhealthy movement habits. This is the opposite of moving youthfully! If a movement is uncomfortable, make it smaller and slower. If you feel strain in your neck while lying down, put a folded towel or two under your head. If it is uncomfortable to lie on your back with your legs long, try placing a rolled-up blanket under your knees or bend your knees and stand your feet on the floor.

You can also modify the position of your body. For example, if the directions call for a straight arm and that is uncomfortable for you, bend your arm slightly. Or, if raising your right arm causes pain, raise your left arm, reversing all of my directions accordingly. It's important that the movements feel pleasant. Think "no pain, *more* gain"!

Small, Slow Movements Equal Big Improvements

Gentle movements done with attention allow you to feel more than large or fast ones. The more you feel, the more your brain can rewire itself. So please don't stretch or strain! Let your movements feel light and easy, and you'll feel younger faster.

Breathe Easily

It is very common for people to hold their breath when they are doing something unusual or challenging. Notice if you have a habit of holding your breath. Allow yourself to breathe in an easy, relaxed way.

Rest Frequently

It is important to take frequent rest breaks when doing these exercises. Even though the movements are not strenuous, you may be using muscles that you have not used in a long time. You will also need to rest your attention, as it is challenging to stay fully attentive for long periods. Rest breaks allow you to "download" your new youthful movement into your nervous system so you can carry it over into your everyday life.

Embrace Novelty

Moving non-habitually creates flexible bodies and minds. Don't simply repeat the movement as if you were doing "reps" at the gym. Instead, change something about *how* you do each movement. For example, find ways to reduce tension around your eyes, jaws, fingers and toes. Where else can you let go of tension? How can the movement be easier and more pleasant? How can you make the movement lighter and easier?

Use Your Imagination

Did you know that when you imagine doing something, you use many of the same parts of your brain as when you actually do it? Use your senses when you imagine moving and you'll gain many (and sometimes more!) of the benefits that you would if you were actually moving. This is especially important when pain, disability or your environment prevent you from moving. Imagine your movement as easy and elegant.

Are You Really Comfortable?

I use the word *comfort* a lot in this book. I suggest, time and again, that you use comfort as your guide in moving yourself and your dog. But many people have lost the ability to sense their comfort. They are so used to *discomfort* that it's become their norm. They may think they're comfortable when it simply feels *familiar*.

Unfortunately, our culture is bombarded with admonitions to "Just do it" despite discomfort. We are told, "No pain, no gain." But the nervous system cannot focus on learning when it is busy defending against pain. Conversely, comfort and pleasure guide the nervous system to discover healthier ways to move. If you have been conditioned to associate comfort with laziness, I would suggest you think of comfort in a new light. I like what Dr. Moshe Feldenkrais said, *"Assertiveness is the ability to discern finer and finer grades of comfort."* What a novel and healthy way to think about being assertive!

The best way to sense your comfort is with slow, small movements done with a quiet mind. This will allow you to notice where you are using effort unnecessarily. If you discover that you are breathing in a shallow, restricted way, you are probably not comfortable. Instead, move lightly and easily. *Find a way to make the movement pleasurable.* Breathe fully as you learn to recognize, and savor, comfort.

Key Points of Chapter One

- Our potential to improve is not limited by age or physical condition, but by the quality of our *attention*. Improved functioning can occur at any life stage.

- Novel movements produce new neural connections, resulting in freer, more comfortable movement.

- Rhythm may stimulate the healing process.

- Paying attention while doing slow, easy movements can yield improved coordination and youthful vitality.

- Exploring variations helps you improve even more.

- Don't settle for *familiar*. Insist on *comfort*.

Chapter Two: A Healing Connection Helps an Older Dog Walk Again

Do you know a dog who can no longer jump in the car or on the bed? Maybe the dog is not very old, but you've noticed that running and jumping are not easy for him anymore. Or maybe your dog still enjoys chasing tennis balls in the park, but she is stiff and sore the next day. Over time, some dogs' hindquarters get so weak that it becomes difficult for them to even walk. Lots of people, too, have trouble going up and down stairs, travelling over uneven ground or simply walking a long distance.

While some may view this as an unavoidable consequence of aging, I have seen many dogs and humans regain their ability to use their legs easily and comfortably. Whether you or your dog have already lost some mobility or you wish to *avoid* this loss, I hope the following story helps set you on the path to moving easier and feeling younger.

Rocky Improves – And So Do I

Listening with your hands can relax a dog and prepare him for improved mobility.

Rocky, an eleven-year-old Australian Shepherd, entered my office on a sunny December afternoon. He was dragging his hind legs, stumbling as he made his way toward me. This beautiful dog was accompanied by Bob, a tall, fit gentleman whose current occupation as a yoga instructor followed a successful career as a high-tech entrepreneur.

After having explored his dog's medical options, Bob brought Rocky to me. He hoped that I could help his aging dog regain stability in his hind legs so that he could walk with greater ease. And if Rocky's walking improved enough, they could go on their annual camping trip to Montana, something that Bob looked forward to each year.

Bob's blue eyes danced as he spoke about the fun that he and Rocky had on these yearly Montana outings. Bob loved connecting with nature as he camped in the forest with his loyal canine companion by his side. He delighted in watching Rocky relish the smells, sounds and sights of the wintry woodland, every sense tingling in doggie delight. And while Bob knew that it was unlikely that he and Rocky would go on a long forest hike again, he hoped that Rocky's walking would improve enough so that he could share at least one more Montana campsite with him.

The long and short of it is that Bob and Rocky did go on their much-anticipated trip. But something besides improved movement happened during our time together. And it happened to me.

The short stroll from the car to my office had been an effort for Rocky, causing him to pant heavily. I invited the Australian Shepherd to lie down on the comfortable mat I kept in my office and he did so readily. I softly settled my hands on his ribcage, letting my hands passively move up and down in time with his breath. I made no attempt to change his breathing. Since my contact was comforting and observant, rather than controlling, it helped Rocky feel safe with me. He soon began to relax.

Novel movements enhance body awareness. The more parts a dog feels, the more he can use.

When Rocky's breathing deepened and slowed, I began gently exploring his body. Slowly and rhythmically, my fingertips gently traced along the length of his spine, delicately lifting a small section of back muscle for a second or two before moving on. These gentle, non-habitual movements felt very different than petting, so they captured

Rocky's attention and helped him become aware of *all* the parts of his spine.

Many animals, including humans, have an incomplete awareness of their bodies. They are often *very* aware of the parts that are overused and hurting, but they tune out other areas. This leads to unbalanced movement, with some parts working harder than others. Over time, this extra wear and tear can lead to stiff, arthritic joints and weakened muscles. Like so many senior dogs, Rocky's body bore the evidence of unbalanced movement.

By drawing attention to his back with my light fingertip movements, I was helping Rocky become aware of *all* the parts of his spine and reminding him that the parts he had been "tuning out" could move too. **I wanted him to *feel* more, so that he could *use* more**. Using more parts would distribute the effort across a greater area, thus reducing the strain on the dog's joints and muscles and improving his balance. After working my way up the other side of his spine, I paused for a moment, giving Rocky's nervous system time to register this key information.

Gratitude bridges the interspecies communication gap.

As I moved to sit cross-legged behind Rocky's tail, I appreciated that this wonderful being put himself, quite literally, "in my hands." As with all the individuals I encounter, I wanted to do everything I could to help him live the best life possible.

I supported Rocky's lower back between my hands, feeling gratitude for the dog and the moment. Rocky took a wonderfully deep breath. As he did so, I felt an intense heat in my heart, unlike anything I had experienced before. It was exhilarating and filled me with a profound sense of well-being and peace. It was the feeling of bliss, pure and simple.

Continuing to work with Rocky, there were times when I would support or move a part of Rocky's body and the warm, delicious feeling in my heart would grow. I could, quite literally, feel the dog's relief. Rocky's deepened breaths validated this impression, and I was thrilled to realize that I was so tuned into Rocky that my heart resonated with him.

While a dog is lying down, you can improve his ability to stand and walk.

With Rocky still lying comfortably on his right side, I covered a three-foot-long foam roller (often sold as a "noodle" pool toy) with a plushy bath towel and placed it under Rocky's left front and hind legs. As I gently rolled the roller, it passively moved Rocky's top-lying legs. My other hand touched specific places on Rocky's back, pelvis and ribcage, reminding him that if these parts moved, the movement of his legs would be easier.

Keeping Rocky on his side allowed him to experience many of the sensations involved in standing and walking, but none of the effort and discomfort that working against gravity created. It was essential that I give his nervous system an experience of walking that involved only comfort and confidence. *But to get Rocky's brain to associate my hands-on movements with walking, I needed to include as many sensations of standing and walking as I could.* The roller between his legs kept his legs about the same width they would be if he were walking in a balanced way.

One at a time, Bob held a very small hardcover book against each of his dog's paws, so that Rocky's brain could register that he was, in effect, "standing" on a firm, flat surface. Even though Rocky was lying on his side, this *"Artificial Floor"* gave Rocky the *sensory* experience of standing. This could stimulate his brain to evoke the physical functions that would allow the Australian Shepherd to stand more easily.

At the same time, I used my hands to passively move parts of the dog's body in a rhythm similar to walking. These were all physical sensations associated with walking, but without the strain and distress. The comfortable sensations served as messages to the dog's brain, indicating that easier walking was a possibility. I hoped this would generate the creation of new neural connections that would improve Rocky's ability to actually stand and walk.

Gently supporting the dog in various places can remind him to use those body parts more efficiently as he walks.

After working with Rocky on both sides, I asked him to stand up. I placed one hand on his back and the other on the underside of his chest. Supporting Rocky with my hands, I shifted his weight in a small circle, moving his mass from one paw to another, with each paw bearing more weight for an instant. We explored shifting his weight from side-to-side and forward and back, too.

As I let my hands go, I could see that standing was easier for Rocky. He was balanced more evenly, with all his toes in contact with the floor. His hind legs were under his body to better support his weight.

As Bob encouraged Rocky to walk around the office, I put my hands on various places of the dog's body, reminding him that these places could participate in the motions involved in walking.

Whereas tight turns used to cause Rocky to fall, he was now able to maneuver around my office in a balanced way. And since his hind legs were now doing more of the work, Rocky no longer had to strain excessively with his front legs and shoulders. His movement was easier and more comfortable. Smiling, Bob called it a "huge improvement." They were going camping after all!

A heart-centered connection enhances the benefits to your dog.

While the movement strategies I employed were crucial to Rocky's improvement, it was clear that the depth of our connection facilitated the successful result. My work, and indeed my life, changed forever on that day. This profound experience taught me the importance of consciously creating an empathic heart connection at the start.

In order to teach others how to create this powerful heart connection with their dog, I developed an exercise called *Connected Breathing.*

Connected Breathing

Listen to the audio recording of *Connected Breathing* by going to www.debonomoves.com/dog-book and typing in the password *free.*

Connected Breathing can create a powerful connection with your dog. It can also help center and ground you in the present moment and generate a feeling of well-being in both canine and human. *Connected Breathing* increases the effectiveness of the other *Debono Moves*.

Benefits may include:

- Relaxes and reduces stress in canine and human.
- Creates a powerful heart-to-heart connection between you and your dog.
- Opens up a channel of communication between you and your dog.
- Enhances feelings of peace and well-being at any life stage or condition.

Find a quiet time and place with a minimum of distractions so that you and your dog can focus on each other as you enjoy the exercise.[8]

Position: Dog lying down.

Practice with your dog. With your dog lying down quietly on his side, sit behind him so that you are facing his back. If your dog would rather not lie on his side at the moment, allow him to choose another position. If sitting on the floor is not comfortable for you, sit on a large pillow or rolled up blanket to help relieve strain on your hips. Alternatively, you can place your dog on a couch or bed and you can sit on a chair before him. You can also sit next to your dog on a sofa or bed. Remember that your comfort is important when doing *Debono Moves,* so please check in with yourself as you work with your dog. If you are uncomfortable, adjust your position to afford yourself maximum comfort and ease of movement.

*If it is impossible for you to get comfortable right next to your dog, you can still do Connected Breathing. Simply sit on a chair or sofa, and when you get to the part where I suggest that you put your hands on your dog, simply **imagine** that your hands are lightly resting on your dog.*

Don't touch your dog yet, but simply sit near him and focus your attention on yourself. How are you breathing? What parts of yourself move as you breathe? Your ribs? Your belly? Your back? Your sides? Do you feel centered and relaxed? If distracting thoughts enter your mind, just let them float on by. Don't judge them, or yourself. Instead, breathe comfortably and take a few moments to notice your physical sensations. Then follow the steps below:

---

[8] If your dog finds it difficult to lie still and relax next to you, please read "How to Help an Anxious or Distracted Dog" in Chapter Six. Additionally, you can do the meditation alone at first. But don't be surprised if your dog soon decides that lying still next to you is a very nice thing to do!

1. Put your attention on the area of your heart, around the center of your chest. You may put a hand on your heart if this helps focus your attention.

2. Breathe in a relaxed way, imaging that the air is coming into and going out of your heart area.

3. Feel the love you have for your dog. Let the feelings of love and appreciation fill your heart.

Consider that the breath you exhale becomes part of the air that your dog inhales. Your dog's exhalations then are mixed with the air you breathe in. And yet air is only a fraction of the unseen that we share with our dogs. The energy of our emotions, for example, affects our animals in many ways. That is why generating positive feelings, such as love or appreciation, matters so much to our dogs. And those positive feelings help us to be happier and healthier as well.

4. As you enjoy feeling grateful for your dog, remember that your dog loves you too. Imagine that the air you inhale is infused with love from your canine friend. Visualize that the air enters your heart area, then lights up every cell in your body.

5. As you exhale, imagine your breath going out through your heart, transmuting it into beautifully-colored light that flows down your arms and out your hands, sending your love back to your dog. Visualize this love lighting up every cell of your dog. You are both radiant beings, filled with shared love and healing light.

Consider how soothing turquoise waves wash up on a beautiful beach. A wave comes in; then it goes back out to the ocean. The ocean would soon lose its power and majesty if the waves never returned. Love is like that too. Your power develops from both sending and receiving love, yet too often we get so busy caring for our loved ones that we forget to nourish ourselves with their love and appreciation for us. We need those waves to be both coming onto the beach as well as going back out, so don't forget to take in the waves of love from your dog! Let those waves wash over you and relax and comfort you.

6. As you maintain this breath connection with your dog, lightly put the palms of your hands on your dog's ribcage, with your hands slightly apart from one another. If your dog is very small, you can place one hand on his ribs and the other lightly on his hindquarters.

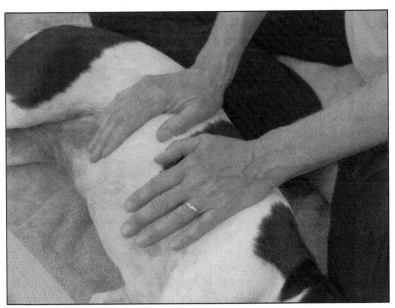

My hands are lightly resting on Ruby's ribcage.

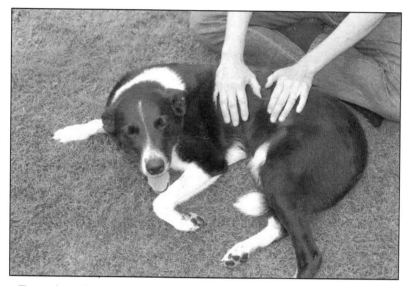

Even though Maggie is not totally relaxed yet, I begin *Connected Breathing.* If you remain patient and calm, most dogs will soon relax and flop onto their side.

7. Feel the continuous rise and fall of your dog's ribcage. Sense how your hands are passively moved in time to your dog's breathing. Remember to keep your hands light. Don't press down or make any other attempt to influence him with your hands.

*Keep in mind that your dog knows the difference between a listening touch and a corrective one. It is the **listening** touch that we wish to develop in Debono Moves. I have found that the more we humans listen to our dogs, the more our dogs listen and respond to us.*

Notice any changes in your dog's – and your own – breathing. What parts of you move as you breathe? Is your breathing slower or faster than when you started? Be mindful of any images or thoughts that spontaneously occur to you. Many people become more "tuned in" to their dog through *Connected Breathing* because its emphasis on listening and

28

"not-doing" helps open up a channel of communication between you and your dog.

As long as both you and your dog are comfortable, you can spend as much time as you'd like enjoying this close connection. You can also put your hands on other parts of your dog's body. While we generally start *Connected Breathing* with the ribcage, your canine may appreciate a supporting hand on his hip and one on his shoulder blade. Or two hands on his back. Or one on his back and one on his chest. Try various places on your dog's body and notice where your dog seems to welcome your quiet hands. Make sure you maintain your comfort and ease throughout. When either you or your dog want to get up, you can simply take your hands off your dog while you maintain the feeling of gratitude.

Even a few minutes of *Connected Breathing* can be healing for you and your dog. Many people start with three to five minutes and progress to longer sessions as they gain experience with the exercise. The more consistently you practice *Connected Breathing*, the more healing benefits you and your canine companion will derive from it. Just remember to relax and enjoy the experience and don't worry about trying to get it "right" or keeping track of the time. Simply feeling love and gratitude is enough.

And while *Connected Breathing* is an effective and complete process on its own, it is also a good starting point for doing other *Debono Moves* with your dog. The quiet, heart-centered connection you create with *Connected Breathing* increases the effectiveness of subsequent *Debono Moves.*

Mary's Tip:

If you are stressed, *Connected Breathing* is a great way to change your emotional state. But what if your dog isn't

nearby? Fortunately, you can still benefit from this exercise. As you follow the steps of *Connected Breathing,* simply visualize your dog breathing with you. Can you imagine what your dog feels like as you softly place your hands on her ribcage and breathe together? You may be surprised at how this exercise can relax and refresh you. *Connected Breathing* not only deepens the human-canine bond, but it can reduce your stress. Try it when you are waiting in line at the grocery store or if you are having trouble falling asleep.

Many people experience a spiritual con-nection with their animal companions that does not diminish over time and space. It can be comforting and healing for grieving people to experience *Connected Breathing* while visualizing their departed dog sharing love and light with them.

The Healing Power of Connection

Does your dog make you smile even when you've had a rough day? Or *especially* when you've had a rough day?

Connecting with a canine is a soul-satisfying kind of joy. They love us unconditionally. Dogs don't care if we haven't styled our hair or organized the garage. They just want to be with us. And we want to be with them.

The human-canine bond not only feels good, it's good for your health too. When you turn off the mind chatter and tune into your dog, you can experience a profound sense of well-being. In the book, *A General Theory of Love,* the term *limbic resonance* is explained as "a symphony of mutual and internal adaptation whereby **two mammals become attuned to each other's inner states**" (*emphasis mine*). The authors write that limbic resonance is "the door to communal connection."[9] It was limbic resonance that helped me sense what Rocky was feeling. I've found it to be a blissful and mutually healing state, as profound and beneficial as deep meditation. Doing *Debono Moves* with your dog can help you attain this depth of connection.

When you are in limbic resonance with your dog, there is no past or future to fret about. You are in present moment awareness. You are in the *now,* a place that we tend to spend far too little time in.

The present moment is the only place where you can act. It is your place of power. *Connecting with your dog in the now allows you to tap into an energy that is greater than yourself, creating a wellspring of healing, hope and love.*

Join your dog in the *now. Debono Moves* can help you get there.

Human Exercise #1: Deeper Breath, Lighter Hands

Benefits: This exercise can help you discover a more efficient way to breathe, which may improve stamina and reduce stress. This exercise also guides you to lighter, more refined use of your hands, freeing you of unnecessary tension and improving your ability to use *Debono Moves* to help your dog.

Listen to the audio recording of this exercise by going to www.debonomoves.com/dog-book and typing in the password *free.*

The exercise is printed and illustrated in Chapter Eight.

---

[9] *A General Theory of Love* is a book about human emotion, authored by Thomas Lewis, Fari Amini and Richard Lannon.

Getting to Know Your Dog in a New Way

I imagine that you stroke and pet your dog quite often, an activity that you probably both enjoy. This exercise will be a bit different, but should be just as pleasurable. You'll explore your dog in a way that helps you learn more about your dog's anatomy *and* can enhance your dog's body awareness. But don't worry, you won't need to memorize any anatomical terms!

Pick a time when your dog is relaxed and you are not in a rush. This process should not be hurried. Think of it like a learning meditation. Or imagine that you are a sculptor who wants to really know what your dog feels like so that you can recreate her canine body as a work of art. Take your time to feel the contours of your dog's body and keep your touch light and gentle. Remember, *the softer your hand, the more you will feel.*

As always, be mindful of your dog's comfort. Explore your dog gently, safely and respectfully.

Position: Dog lying on her side.

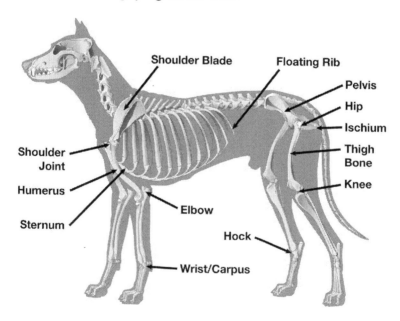

The Front Leg

With your dog lying on her side, put your hand gently on her front paw. Slowly slide your hand up your dog's leg just a little bit until you get to the first part that bends. This is the dog's *carpus* or wrist. Slide your hand farther up and you'll come to your dog's *elbow*.

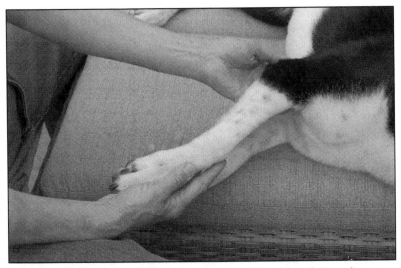

The index finger of my right hand is touching Maggie's wrist area. My left hand is holding her elbow.

The bone that connects the elbow to the shoulder blade is called the *humerus*. You may notice that canine anatomy has a lot of similarities to human anatomy. Slide your hand up the humerus until it is close to your dog's chest.

The Shoulder Blade

Keep sliding your soft hand up your dog's leg. Can you feel where your dog's front leg attaches to her shoulder blade? The shoulder blade is also called the *scapula*. Using your fingertips, trace the outline of her shoulder blade. Do you feel how it angles backward a bit? The shoulder blade moves forward and back in response to movements of the forelegs. As the front leg reaches forward, the top of the shoulder blade moves back. And as the front leg goes backward, the top of the shoulder blade tips forward. You can gently pick up your dog's front leg and do a very small movement of taking the leg forward and backward. Can you see and feel the shoulder blade moving?

Look at the illustration of the skeleton to see how some of your dog's ribs lie under the shoulder blade. The shoulder blade glides over these ribs. Dogs don't have clavicles (collar bones), so there is no bony attachment of the shoulder blade to the rest of the body. It is held in place by soft tissue, including ligaments and muscles.

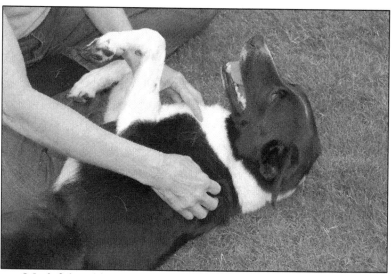

My left hand is touching the *shoulder joint.* My right hand touches the top of Maggie's *shoulder blade.*

The Ribs

Place your hands on your dog's ribcage. Dogs have 13 pairs of ribs. Can you find the last rib on each side? On some dogs, these short ribs are quite prominent. How many ribs can you feel on your dog?

The costal cartilages of the first nine pairs of ribs articulate with the *sternum*. The costal cartilages of the next three pairs of ribs attach to adjacent costal cartilages, forming the *costal arch*. The 13th pair of ribs are the *floating ribs*, since they are not attached to sternal cartilage. They are at the very back of the ribcage.

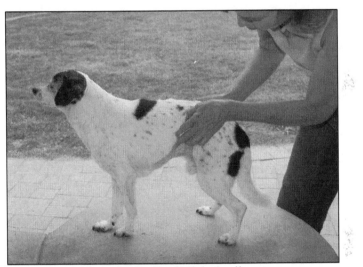

This is the back of Nicky's ribcage.

The Sternum

Place your hand softly on the front of your dog's chest. Can you feel a bone right in the middle? This bone is called the *sternum*, or breastbone. Can you find the very top of this bone? This top piece is called the *manubrium*. Use your fingertips to trace the sternum down its length. Find the end of the sternum, which is located on your dog's underside, near the abdomen. This last part is called the *xiphoid process.*

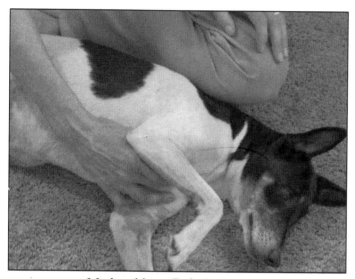

My hand is on Ruby's sternum.

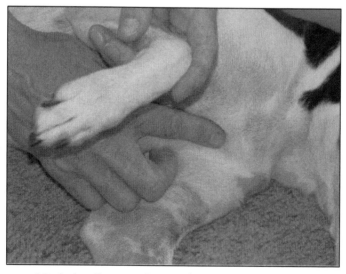

My index finger points to the top of the sternum.

The Spine

Your dog's spine starts where the first neck vertebrae joins the skull; it continues through the middle of your dog's back, and it ends in the last bony part of your dog's tail. Use your fingers to slowly trace the entire length of your dog's spine. How much of your dog's spine can you feel? Notice the shape of the first two neck vertebrae.

The dog's spine has 7 cervical (neck) vertebrae, 13 thoracic vertebrae, 7 lumbar, 3 sacral (fused in adults to form the *sacrum)* and about 20 coccygeal (tail) vertebrae, although this last number can vary a great deal between dogs. There are often variations in the exact number of spinal vertebrae. For example, some dogs have six, rather than seven, lumbar vertebrae.

The Hind Leg

Place your hand on your dog's hind paw. Slowly run your hand up your dog's leg until you come to the first angle, which is called the *hock.* This is somewhat similar to our ankle joint. Continue sliding your hand up the leg until you come to the next angle, which is the dog's knee, or *stifle.* The bone that connects the knee to the hip is called the *femur* or thigh bone. Can you feel this bone?

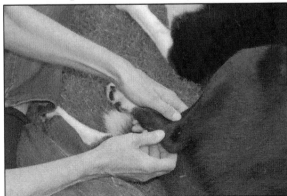

The *hock* is similar to our ankle.

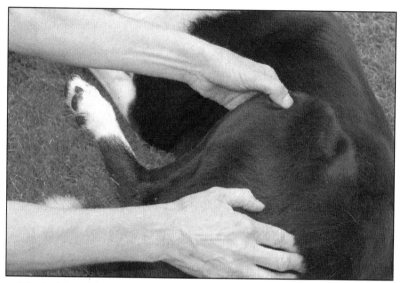

My left hand is on Maggie's *stifle,* which is similar to our knee.
My right hand is on the outside of her *hip joint.*

The Hip Joint

Keep one hand on the thigh bone. Look at the illustration
of the dog skeleton and estimate where your dog's *hip joint*
may be. Put your second hand in that spot. With the first hand
that is lightly holding the thigh bone, very gently move the leg
forward and backward a little. Notice if you feel movement
under your second hand. Move this hand around until you can
feel a slight movement. When you do, you've found the hip
joint!

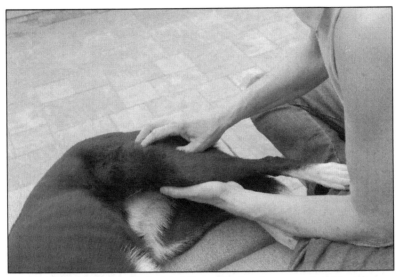

As I support Maggie's thigh bone, I slowly move her hind leg forward and back. My right hand feels the subtle movement in the *hip joint.*

The Ischium

Put your hands on the very back of your dog's pelvis, right below the tail. Put one hand on the right and one on the left. Can you feel those bones that stick out? Those are the dog's *ischia.*

There is a right *ischium* and a left *ischium.* Feel their shape and size.

We have ischia too. In humans, they are often referred to as "sit bones," "seat bones," also known as "sitz bones."

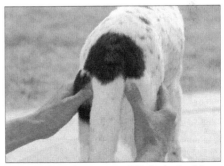

My thumbs are on Nicky's ischia.

The Head

Make your way up to your dog's head. Use your fingertips to delicately trace around your dog's skull. Feel the contours and ridges of your dog's head. Notice where the skull meets the spine.

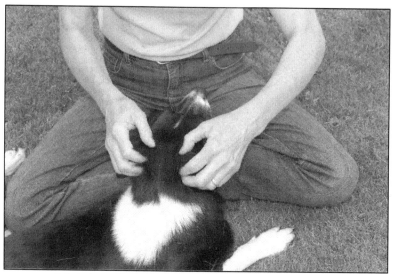

Maggie enjoys my gentle exploration of her head.

Now that you've explored your dog's body, can you imagine what your dog's skeleton looks like under all that fur? This exercise not only improves your knowledge of your dog's anatomy, but it can help *enhance your dog's body awareness* too.

When I'm doing *Debono Moves,* I find it useful to visualize the skeleton of the dog I'm working with. I hope this exercise helps you know your dog a little bit better.

Human Exercise #2: Improve Your Walking by Lying Down

Benefits: Just as the recumbent Rocky improved his walking, you can too! This relaxing exercise contains movements that occur when you walk. By doing the movements while lying down, you can harness the power of your brain to learn how to walk more easily and efficiently. More comfortable walking reduces wear and tear damage and can help you feel more youthful!

Listen to the audio recording of this exercise by going to www.debonomoves.com/dog-book and typing in the password *free.*

The exercise is printed and illustrated in Chapter Eight.

Key Points of Chapter Two

- Listening with your hands can relax a dog and prepare him for improved mobility.
- Novel movements enhance body awareness. The more parts a dog feels, the more he can use.
- The softer you touch, the more you can feel.
- Gratitude bridges the interspecies communication gap.
- While a dog is lying down, you can improve his ability to stand and walk.
- Gently supporting the dog in various places can remind him to use those body parts more efficiently as he walks.
- A heartfelt connection deepens the effectiveness of hands-on work.

- The human-canine bond not only feels good, it's good for your health too.
- Connecting with your dog allows you to tap into an energy that is greater than yourself, creating a wellspring of healing, hope and love.

Chapter Three: Improved Back Flexibility Got These Dogs Moving Again

Have you ever strained your back? Or felt stiffness in your spine? Whether you walk on two legs or four, back problems are a fact of life for many of us, especially as we get older. But limitations in the back don't always show up as problems in the spine. They may appear as muscle strains or other difficulties with the legs. The following two dogs had very different symptoms: the first dog, a shaggy white Spinone mix named Cassie, kept collapsing on walks, and her vet diagnosed her with severe spinal arthritis. The second dog, a brown Boxer named Oti, had a hamstring muscle strain that was taking a long time to heal.

Interestingly, both of these dogs improved when I helped them use their backs more freely. And the same is often true with humans. Stiffness and achiness often arises from over-using some parts of our spine and underusing others. Whether you are dealing with back strain, arthritis or tight hamstrings, or wish to avoid these problems, the following chapter may help you and your dog move more freely into your golden years.

Cassie Overcomes Spinal Arthritis

The following was written by Cassie's "mom," Michele McDougal.

My boyfriend and I adopted this shaggy, white, 70-pound Spinone mix 2-1/2 years ago. Among other passions, our Cassie is a "squirrel girl." The highlight of her existence is our daily walk in the park; and she is in hunting mode from the moment her paws hit the ground. In May 2001, her fixation on squirrels almost did her in. After having pulled the leash right out of my hand, she was in the heat of what a friend called a "blind run," a full-speed pursuit of a squirrel who was inside the fencing of a baseball diamond. She simply didn't see the chain link fence that separated her from her prey until it was too late. Although I couldn't see it from my vantage point, I heard her hit the fence full force – it was a horrible sound.

At first she seemed a little stunned, but otherwise okay. As we made our way home, her usual, seemingly-effortless trot slowed to a walk; her head lowered; and then she dropped down on the pavement. It was hot and she was tired, so I hoped that was the reason for her behavior. After a few minutes I coaxed her up and we slowly walked home. Upon our arrival, she plopped down on the living room floor, and this time she didn't get back up.

Cassie is my first dog and her "dad" was out of town, so I did what any mother would do. I panicked and then we headed to our veterinarian. The first thing the doctor did was gently cup Cassie's muzzle in his hands and lift her lips to examine her mouth, something I never would have thought to do, and found her gums to be shredded and bloody. He surmised that she hit the fence head first and followed up his examination with some X-rays.

Thankfully there were no spinal fractures or other internal injuries. He gave her a shot of something for the pain and sent us home with pain pills. The next day Cassie seemed fine.

A few days later, however, down she went again, and once again, she couldn't get up. Off to the vet we went and this time he X-rayed her back and hips. "There's our problem!" he declared. He pointed to the X-ray where he identified large arthritic lesions in her lumbar spine. He also informed me, considering the advanced state of her arthritis, that our Cassie had to be two or three years older than we had been told when we adopted her. Our option was singular: surgery; very expensive and very risky. My vet cautioned that her condition would get progressively worse and it would soon be obvious when we'd need to schedule the procedure.

Because of her "new age," and given the empirical evidence on film, we accepted the diagnosis; but surgery was the last thing we wanted for our baby. And it was indeed risky. She could wind up incontinent and/or with paralysis. There was no way we were going to wait for this eventuality! Meanwhile, Cassie's episodes of falling and staying down ramped up from an average of once per month to once a week. We were frightened.

We began a long process of investigating and trying alternative approaches, including massage, Reiki, acupuncture, veterinary orthopedic manipulation, and Chinese herbal remedies – we even consulted an interspecies communicator to see if Cassie herself could tell us anything about her condition! Then we found Mary Debono.

Mary saw Cassie only three times; and after the second visit, she said that she didn't think Cassie needed her anymore. It was I who insisted that we needed to see Mary at least one more time! I don't know exactly what Mary does except that *Debono Moves,* which Mary developed, helps the animal choose other options for movement, retraining the body's habits. I do know that it was a struggle for her dad and me to stay awake during the sessions because there was something so peaceful and relaxing, almost spiritual, about the experience. Cassie thought so too.

We are now within days of having four full months without a single event – the longest period since her accident. Last week, I watched Cassie run full speed ahead, leash free, on a Northern California beach. My heart soared at the sight!

I can't thank Mary Debono enough for the work she did to perfect *Debono Moves.*

Mary Writes About Cassie

Injuries and arthritis can occur when body parts are habitually overstressed.

When Cassie came to my office, she was dealing with two traumas, one acute and one chronic. The acute trauma came when she hit the fence at full speed. The chronic trauma was the arthritis in her lower spine.

Cassie was seemingly asymptomatic before her accident. Her arthritis, although classified as "advanced," had been hidden just below the level of awareness. It took a headlong gallop into a fence to bring it up to the surface, causing Cassie, and those who loved her, some real problems.

Cassie, however, had been coping with her arthritis long before she met the fence. It is likely that her nervous system had already altered her movement patterns to compensate for the discomfort and stiffness caused by the arthritic lesions. All of this can go on without it being obvious to anyone. After all, Cassie was a relatively young dog, full of life, running and playing with abandon.

Many times arthritis develops because the individual overuses a particular part of the body. The reason a part gets overused is because other parts are not doing their share of the work. Cassie had arthritis in the area where the lumbar vertebrae meet the sacrum. This place, commonly referred to as the "L/S joint," is capable of much movement, so it's easy for the body to let this part work hard while the other parts of the spine are tuned out. And when some parts are left out of a movement, other parts have to work harder than nature intended. Those parts can sustain wear and tear damage.

Once arthritis develops, the nervous system inhibits movement to minimize the pain. While it is an effective short-term strategy, this lack of movement creates a vicious cycle, leading to greater strain on joints and muscles. My job was to help Cassie interrupt this vicious cycle and hopefully lessen the chance of her arthritis causing her any more problems.

Help the dog relax first.

To start the session, Michele asked Cassie to lie on her side. Understandably nervous about what was going to happen, Cassie refused. She was only comfortable lying in the "sphinx" position. Since it is important to keep the animal feeling safe and comfortable in a *Debono Moves* session, we began with Cassie lying like a sphinx.

Cassie was in pain, and a nervous system distracted by pain and tension is incapable of learning. Since such a nervous system is busy defending itself against the threat of more pain, it can't process new sensory information. Therefore, the first step is to quiet the nervous system by eliminating the "background noise" of chronic muscular tension and anxiety.

I used my hands to softly lift the muscles along Cassie's back. As I supported each small area of muscle, Cassie began to relax. Before I knew it, Cassie flopped to her side, obviously confident that no harm would come to her.

In addition to helping her release tense back muscles, the delicate and evenly-paced lifting movements were giving Cassie's nervous system a rhythmic stimulus to organize around. Using rhythm is a wonderful way to quiet the nervous system and increase relaxation. The gentle lifts along her back were also increasing her awareness (and thus her use) of her entire spine. In addition, my actions were showing Cassie that movement was *possible* and comfortable throughout her *whole* back.

With Cassie's nervous system no longer engaged in maintaining its safety or distracted by energy and attention-sapping muscular effort, it could attend to the sensory information being conveyed by my hands.

Awakening the ribs can make it easier to move the spine in a healthy way.

After working with her entire spine from head to tail, I used a fingertip to gently lift the muscle in between two ribs.

This movement induced a sigh of relief from Cassie. I worked my way through Cassie's ribcage, effectively outlining and highlighting all her ribs.

Increasing awareness of the dog's body brings about a greater distribution of effort, thus relieving strain throughout the system. The more parts that participate in a movement, the easier and more elegant the movement becomes.

Thoroughly enjoying the work with her ribcage, Cassie was now close to dozing off. It was my hope that Cassie would use her ribs more effectively since they were now clearer in her body awareness. And since the ribs are directly connected to the mid-back, using the ribs more efficiently is a way to improve the use of the back.

Connecting the pieces of the body promotes healthier, coordinated movement.

After working with Cassie on both sides, I placed one hand gently on her head and my other hand against the back end of her pelvis. I gently pushed through her pelvis, seeing a wave of movement travel from her hind end all the way to her head. My intent was to have Cassie feel the relationship between her head and her hind end. This would allow her to notice, and thus to use, all the parts in between. I removed my hand from her head and placed it on her sternum, or chest bone. As I pressed through her pelvis, I was again giving Cassie the sensation of connection between her hind end and her front end, this time highlighting the connection between her ribcage and pelvis.

Since the *Debono Moves* were pleasurable, Cassie's nervous system would want to recreate them on her own. In other words, she could learn to use her whole back more fully after experiencing how easy and enjoyable the new movement felt. From her *Debono Moves* sessions, Cassie's nervous system had created a new "body map." This new image more accurately reflected the movements her body was capable of.

As a result, Cassie immediately began to use her back in a fuller, more efficient way. She was now unstuck from her habitual ways of moving. And she could once again run and play without pain.

Recovering from a Chronic Muscle Injury

Otis. The name alone conjures up an image of a big, happy dog. And Otis, or *Oti* as he was commonly called, fit that image. With a penchant for jumping up and enthusiastically licking unsuspecting visitors, the brown Boxer exuded joy from every pore.

But this cheerful dog had a problem. He was lame on his right hind leg and moved stiffly, especially when he arose from a nap. His veterinarian diagnosed a soft tissue injury, most likely a hamstring strain. He advised Oti's guardians to keep Oti as quiet as possible during the healing process. And then he reassured them that their dog would be back to normal fairly quickly.

But several weeks later, Oti was still limping. He was particularly stiff when he got up each morning. This was worrisome, but the vet couldn't find anything wrong beyond the hamstring strain. Saddened to see their beloved boy still in pain, Oti's people enlisted my help to support their dog's recovery.

Upon meeting Oti, I noticed that the Boxer's left hind leg was significantly more developed than his right hind leg, indicating that he had been compensating for the painful right side for a long time. The hamstrings on both hind legs were quite tight. Taut muscles, of course, are more likely to become injured.

Tight hamstrings often arise from a tight back.

While many people might expect me to focus on the strained muscle, I didn't do that, since focusing on the injured area seldom resolves the underlying problem. Because I know that tight hamstrings often arise from a tight back, I used my hands to gently explore Oti's spine and surrounding muscles. The Boxer was lying on his side as I did this. Not surprisingly, his back was quite tense.

Remember the childhood song, *"Dem Bones"*? It includes phrases such as *"The hip bone is connected to the leg bone."* That song often comes to mind when I work. And while some of these bony connections are obvious, there are others that are not. For instance, there is a strong connection between your ribcage and spine. When movements of your ribcage become freer, your spine is better able to move too.

Moving the ribcage can help relax the back.

With this connection in mind, I put one hand on the underside of the Boxer's ribcage and gently moved his sternum and ribs. My other hand rested lightly on his lower back so that I could feel how the movements of his ribcage created a very subtle rounding of his lower back, which helped release the tension in his back muscles. Holding my hand on his lower back helped the dog feel this too. Oti, relaxed by these gentle movements, fell asleep.

Connecting different body parts through movement can improve coordination.

I removed my hand from the Boxer's lower back and slid it under his pelvis. Using small, delicate movements, I brought his pelvis and ribcage a little closer together. And then I moved them away from each other. These easy, light movements reminded Oti's brain how it could better coordinate his movement.

When the Boxer stood up at the end of our session, his lower back looked noticeably smoother and his hamstrings felt freer. He still had a limp, but his overall movement was more fluid.

Nine days later, I returned to give Oti another *Debono Moves* session, and I was thrilled to see that he had improved dramatically. The Boxer showed only the slightest stiffness upon first getting up after a rest, and he no longer favored his right hind leg. I was confident that even this residual stiffness would soon be a thing of the past. Indeed, it took only another week for it to disappear completely. *Improving the dog's coordination of movement had reduced the strain on his hamstrings and had been the key to his recovery.* With his hamstring no longer unduly stressed, the dog's muscle sprain was able to fully heal.

Human Exercise #3: Easier Sitting

Benefits: Like our canine friends Cassie and Otis, many humans restrict the movement of their spine, which can lead to stiffness and injury. This exercise can help you sit in a way that not only feels better, but can improve the health of your spine.

Sitting more comfortably will also enable you to do *Debono Moves* more easily and effectively with your dog.

Listen to the audio recording of this exercise by going to www.debonomoves.com/dog-book and typing in the password *free.*

The exercise is printed and illustrated in Chapter Eight.

Make It All About You and Your Dog

Sitting on the floor with the German Shepherd lying next to me, I molded my hands around the dog's shoulder. Almost immediately, her breathing deepened and she relaxed. Then suddenly the dog, whose name was Phanta, picked up her head and was on high alert. Speaking in a soothing tone, I helped her unwind again. But after a couple of minutes, the black and tan dog jerked her head up and was on guard. This cycle repeated itself several times. Obviously, something wasn't right.

The dog's human, Rhonda, had an idea. She knew that her dog took her role as defender and guardian seriously, and she wondered if Phanta was unable to relax because I was a stranger. The German Shepherd wasn't as protective of Rhonda's husband Chuck, so we called him into the room and Rhonda left.

Switching humans worked like a charm! As soon as Chuck entered the room, Phanta relaxed. With the distraction of being on guard duty now eliminated, the German Shepherd was able to enjoy a beneficial session that helped her move more comfortably despite her hip dysplasia.

As Phanta demonstrated, the environment plays a role in our ability to help our animals. As you prepare to practice *Debono Moves* with your dog, notice the environment. Does it promote a calm, relaxed state for you and your dog?

Here are some things to consider:

- **Select an appropriate time of day.** If you're asking your dog to lie still and relax when she's usually eating her dinner, you may be asking too much! Reschedule your *Debono Moves* time for when she is satiated and has had some time to relax after her meal. If it's *your* usual dinnertime, you may be unable to fully focus on your dog. Plan accordingly.

- **Expend excess energy.** Has your dog had the opportunity to burn off steam? It's easier for a dog to be still and enjoy your touch when she's recently had the chance to run and play.

- **Minimize distractions.** You can improve the effectiveness of your *Debono Moves* by keeping other dogs, cats, children and uninformed adults away. Find a quiet, comfortable spot in the house or yard where you won't be disturbed.

- **Mind your mental environment.** Turn off your phone and mentally unplug yourself from any concerns. Put your hands on your dog and feel your connection. Breathe. Allow this time to be *all about you and your dog, right now.*

Back Lifts

View a video of Mary teaching *Back Lifts* by going to www.debonomoves.com/dog-book and typing in the password *free*.

Benefits may include:

- Releases back tension and stiffness.
- Relaxes and reduces stress in you and your dog.
- Promotes healthier, more balanced movement.

Position: *Back Lifts* can be done while your dog is lying flat on her side, lying on her chest (like a sphinx), sitting or standing. It's usually easiest to learn the feel of them while your dog is lying down, so we'll start there. Feel free to explore doing *Back Lifts* with your dog in the other positions too.

Practice with your dog. Find a quiet time and place with a minimum of distractions so that you and your dog can focus on each other as you enjoy the exercise.[10]

With your dog lying quietly, sit on the floor behind her tail. If she is lying on her side, you can sit facing her back.

Find the back of your dog's ribs. Place your hands on either side of the spine, just behind your dog's ribcage[11]. Put your thumbs lightly on either side of her spine (the right thumb to the right of her spine, the left thumb to the left of her spine).

Your thumbs should not be on the spine, but about an inch or so away from it. They shouldn't be exerting any pressure, but just lightly rest there. Note that if your dog is lying entirely on her side, you can slide one hand underneath her back. It's helpful to have something soft for you dog to lie on, both for her sake and your own.

You can also do *Back Lifts* with one hand. This can be useful when your dog is lying flat on her side and it's not easy to slip your hand under her.

Your other fingers will be a few inches away from her spine. Distributing the gentle pressure throughout your hand, do a very light lifting motion so that you are gently supporting your dog's soft tissue towards her spine. The lifting movement should be *very small and light.* Think of your hands coming a little bit closer to each other. Remember, this is a *small, light movement.* If your animal shows any discomfort, lighten your contact, or simply stop what you are doing. Most dogs enjoy *Back Lifts.*

---

[10] If your dog finds it difficult to lie still and relax next to you, please read "How to Help an Anxious or Distracted Dog," in Chapter Six.

[11] While I often start *Back Lifts* at the part of the dog's back right in front of the tail, many people find it easier to get the feel of the *Back Lift* when they are on a more "meaty" area of the dog's back, such as the area directly behind your dog's ribcage.

As long as your dog is comfortable, you can hold each lift anywhere from several seconds to about half a minute or so. I suggest that you don't count the time, since the mental activity of counting will reduce your sensitivity. Instead, simply hold the lift through several of your exhalations. *This will also remind you to breathe!*

Release your lift very slowly. Remember that these are small, virtually imperceptible motions. Repeat the lifting motion on the same area a few times, holding it for several seconds to about half a minute each time. After about three lifts in one area, slowly slide your fingers a little bit forward (towards your dog's head) and repeat the *Back Lift.*

Just like you did earlier, lift for several seconds to a minute each time. After two or three lifts in one spot, advance your hands a little bit towards your dog's head and repeat the lifts. Be mindful at all times of your dog's responses, and notice if there are certain places on her back where your dog especially enjoys this support.

I can't emphasize enough that this is a very gentle, light and small movement. Do only what is entirely comfortable for you and your animal.

You can continue moving up your dog's body this way, towards her head. Stop when you reach the back of her shoulder blades. You may go back to her tail and repeat the entire line of *Back Lifts* if you and your dog remain comfortable and interested in these movements.

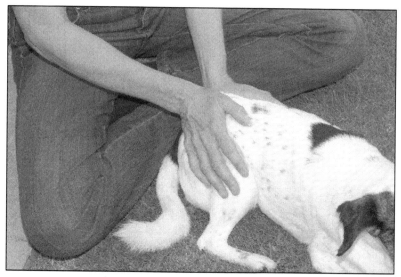

You can start *Back Lifts* on the dog's lower back, in front of the tail.

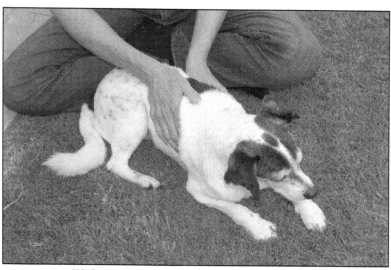

Eighteen-year-old Nicky enjoys *Back Lifts*.

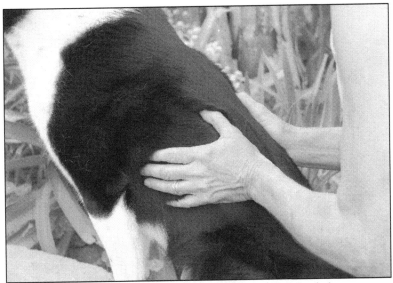

Back Lifts can also be done while your dog is sitting.

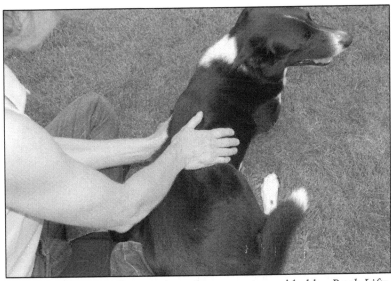

Maggie, like most dogs, enjoys the support provided by *Back Lifts*.

Mary's Tip:

It's essential that you and your dog be comfortable when doing *Debono Moves*. If you are not comfortable sitting on the floor, your dog can be on a low padded table or sofa while you sit in a chair. You can also sit beside your dog on a couch.

Another option is to safely position your dog on a high surface, such as a wall or picnic table, so that you can stand next to your dog. Feel free to come up with other alternatives, always ensuring that you and your dog feel safe and comfortable.

Ribcage Rolls

View a video of Mary teaching *Ribcage Rolls* by going to www.debonomoves.com/dog-book and typing in the password *free*.

Benefits include:

- Releases overall tension and stiffness.
- Helps dog's shoulders move more comfortably.
- Can release stress in dog's back, ribcage and neck.

Position: *Ribcage Rolls* can be done while your dog is lying flat on his side, lying on his chest (like a sphinx), sitting or standing. A nice way to introduce *Ribcage Rolls* is to do them immediately following *Back Lifts*.

Practice with your dog. Do *Back Lifts* from tail to just behind shoulder blades. When your fingers arrive at the back of your dog's shoulder blades, lift the back on one side only. Both hands will remain in contact, but only one hand produces any pressure. Feel how your left hand can gently shift your dog's ribcage slightly to the right. Then feel how your right hand can softly shift her ribcage to the left.

Go back and forth, slowly and softly, rolling your dog's ribcage from side to side. Repeat several times, making sure that your pressure is light and your movements gentle and slow. Do only what is comfortable for you and your dog.

You can move your hands back a little bit and roll your dog's ribcage from various places. As always, stay soft and light and only do what is comfortable for you and your dog.

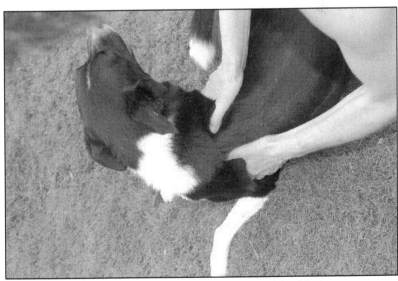

Ribcage Rolls behind Maggie's shoulder blades.

Mary's Tip:

Before you do a *Back Lift, Ribcage Roll* or any other move, put your hands on your dog and simply *imagine* the movement. Imagine doing the movement a couple of times and then make the *smallest* movement you can with your dog.

Do the movement so lightly that someone watching may not see anything, but you and your dog can feel a small, subtle shift. A small, subtle movement is big enough. Keep your hands light and relaxed, and keep this in mind: *small movements can produce big changes.* Big movements, on the other hand, may not be welcomed by your dog.

Human Exercise #4: Lengthen Your Hamstrings Without Stretching

Benefits: Like Otis the Boxer, many people suffer from tight hamstrings. This exercise will help you feel the relationship between your hamstrings and your back. By learning to move your spine freely, you can improve your flexibility and naturally lengthen your hamstrings.

Listen to the audio recording of this exercise by going to www.debonomoves.com/dog-book and typing in the password *free.*

The exercise is printed and illustrated in Chapter Eight.

Key Points of Chapter 3

- Injuries and arthritis can occur when parts of the body are habitually overworked.

- Enhancing body awareness can reduce muscular strain and may lessen the likelihood of injury and arthritis.

- Tight hamstrings often arise from a tight, stiff back.

- A flexible ribcage leads to a flexible back.

- You get the biggest improvement in mobility with a relaxed dog/human.

- Connecting body parts through hands-on movement can improve coordination and balance, leading to healthier movement and full recovery from injury.

- Imagine the movement first, then do the smallest movement you can make.

- Small movements produce big changes.

- For best results, set aside quiet, uninterrupted time to do *Debono Moves* with your dog.

Chapter Four: Getting Rid of a Pain in the Neck

Who hasn't experienced a stiff neck at one time or another? Neck strain is a common occurrence in humans and it often resolves without much intervention. But sometimes a stiff neck is a symptom of a larger problem. You could even be straining your neck a little bit every day, but never enough to experience a "crick in your neck." Since the process is gradual, you may not even notice that you can't turn your head as easily as you once did.

Over time this strain can result in arthritis or other degenerative changes that may produce nerve pain, numbness and/or reduced mobility. Suddenly you realize that it's difficult to look behind you when you're backing out of a parking space. Or maybe you experience a constant feeling of achiness or heaviness in your head and neck. That can make you feel old fast!

Dogs can develop arthritis and other degenerative changes in their necks too. The following chapter explains how I helped a dog regain full use of his neck after an injury. The same strategy can also help your dog to minimize wear and tear damage.

In this chapter you will also learn how to do a *Debono Move* **together** with your dog that can help both of you discover easier, more comfortable movement in your back and neck.

A Neck Injury Doesn't Stop this Canine Athlete

Vicki found her black-and-white dog suddenly unable to pick up his head. The dog, whose name is Nicky, was moving very slowly, holding his head unnaturally low and still. Vicki immediately rushed the 17-pound dog to the veterinarian, who fortunately ruled out a spinal injury. Nicky was diagnosed with a soft tissue injury and prescribed anti-inflammatories and rest. The vet also gave the okay for me to work with Nicky to help him recover fully.

How exactly the dog injured his neck was anyone's guess, but the ten-year-old canine dynamo was often seen jumping off beds, couches and stone walls. Nicky, who was probably a mix of Chihuahua, Cocker Spaniel and Rat Terrier, may have had a collision while roughhousing with one of his larger canine siblings. He also excelled at doing the "zoomies," running in circles at top speed around their expansive back yard. It was this enthusiasm for motion that helped him become a fine canine flyball athlete. Nicky was a bundle of energy and love, and so very irresistible. Vicki didn't have to work hard to convince me to see him as soon as possible.

I had known Vicki, an avid dog lover, for years. I first met the tall, blonde woman when her elderly Australian Shepherd began having issues maintaining his balance and walking. Vicki's home, located just a few minutes from my office, was full of happy, rescued dogs and I always enjoyed going there.

Later that day I pulled my tan Ford Escort up to her coastal home. As I got out of my car, I waved to Vicki's neighbor Bill, who was working on his front lawn. It was nice to see this grey-haired gentleman, whose propensity for carrying dog biscuits made him a veritable celebrity to the neighborhood canines.

I knocked on Vicki's door and was invited in. As I entered her spacious, tiled living room, four dogs of various sizes greeted me. As the black-and-white dogs barked and jumped around me in greeting, I had to laugh. I teased Vicki that she was so coordinated that even her dogs matched! But my smile faded when I realized that Nicky was not among my greeters. It felt odd that the pint-sized dog was not a part of the joyous canine melee that always announced a visitor's arrival. When she saw me looking around for Nicky, Vicki pointed to a corner of the room. There I saw the little short-haired black-and-white dog standing quietly, his head down.

Connecting with the dog is an important first step.

As Vicki ushered her other dogs out of the room, I walked over to Nicky to say hello. Sitting on the floor next to him, I asked him to lie down on his bed. When Nicky rested on his left side, I put my hands ever so gently on his ribcage, feeling the rise and fall of his chest. Taking the time to breathe together helped me create a connection with the little dog. My quiet, listening hands assured Nicky that I wasn't going to cause him discomfort. After a couple of minutes, Nicky's breathing become deeper. So did mine.[12]

Slow, rhythmic movements can be used to stimulate recovery of an injured or anxious dog.

The little dog and I breathed together for several minutes, then I slipped the tips of my right middle and ring fingers into the small space between two of Nicky's ribs. I slowly lifted the soft tissue in a small circle, putting a little bit more pressure on the upward arc of the circle. *The **emphasis on the upward lift** can provide a feeling of relief to sore, tight muscles.* I then slid my fingers up a little bit and made another circle. I circled my way up Nicky's side until I reached the little dog's back. I then repeated this process in the space between an adjacent set of ribs. And then between the next set of ribs, and so on. I made these circles slowly, lightly and rhythmically. Hence their name, *Rhythm Circles.*

The slow, gentle movements relaxed Nicky, interrupting the vicious cycle of pain and anxiety that an injury can create. As I drew *Rhythm Circles* between his ribs, I imagined each

---

[12] To learn this *Connected Breathing* technique, please see Chapter Two.

one becoming a healing vibration that spread out like ripples in a pond. After doing this work for more than 20 years, I have developed a theory about animals that suffer injury, pain or stress. It seems that a single traumatic event, or a series of smaller traumas, can cause some animals to lose the internal rhythm that helps regulate their well-being. I have found that *Rhythm Circles* act like a metronome, providing a slow rhythmic stimulus that the animal uses to reset his rhythm. In cases like this, the change in the dog after doing *Rhythm Circles* can be dramatic. *Rhythm Circles* can be very helpful when there is injury, pain, neuromuscular tension or anxiety.[13]

Non-habitual movements help "wake up" parts of the dog's body, creating more comfortable, balanced movement.

Rhythm Circles feel pleasant and soothing. But they also feel unusual, not at all like the common sensations produced when we pet or scratch our dogs. Since non-habitual experiences stimulate the brain, the *Rhythm Circles* could "wake up" Nicky's ribcage, creating new neural connections between his brain and his ribcage. This would make it more likely that Nicky would use his ribcage to help turn his head, reducing strain on his neck. The less strain the dog experienced, the better the chance that his neck would heal without complications or delay.

Improving the movement of the ribcage can reduce strain in the neck.

I continued making *Rhythm Circles* for about 20 minutes. Then it was time for Nicky to experience how easily his ribcage could now move. Since the ribcage, shoulder and neck are so closely connected, improvements in one part contribute to improvements in the other parts. With the little

---

[13] For another example of the use of rhythmic movements, see Buttons' story in Chapter One.

dog still lying on his left side, I placed my palms lightly on the right side of his ribcage. Nicky and I spent a moment simply breathing together, then I gently slid his ribcage towards his head, holding that position for several seconds. *This was a very small movement that is felt, but not easily seen.* Nicky began to take deeper breaths, which let me know that it was a pleasant sensation and was probably relieving stress in the muscles at the base of his neck. I released my light pressure very gradually, letting his ribcage gently slide back. We repeated these *Ribcage Slides* a few times.

Novel movement combinations help the brain discover easier, healthier movement.

I continued along in this vein, adding in movements of Nicky's right shoulder too. Sometimes I moved his shoulder alone, sometimes with his ribcage. Other times I alternated moving them together, then separately, then together again.[14] *These novel movements could stimulate Nicky's brain to discover easier, healthier movement.*

I then sat behind Nicky's tail and used my hands to help him feel how moving his pelvis could invite movement in his lower back and ribcage. Like a chain, one part of the body affects another. A freely moving neck is dependent on a freely moving ribcage, lower back and pelvis.

Supporting a dog's skeleton can free up the muscles. And change the brain.

Next, my fingers found the two bones at the very back of the dog's pelvis, slightly below the level of the tail. You can easily feel these bones, which together are referred to as

---

[14] See *Shoulder and Ribcage Circles* later in this chapter.

ischia. There is one *ischium* on each side of the pelvis[15]. I placed my hand against Nicky's right ischium, and lightly pressed against the bone. My gentle pressure created a *subtle* wave of movement that traveled from the dog's pelvis to his head. I held this light pressure for several seconds, then released it very gradually. Nicky's breathing deepened each time I did this.

It is easy to understand why Nicky enjoyed this skeletal support. Normally, when a dog wants to move, the nervous system tells muscles to contract. These muscular contractions pull on bones, producing movement. But by gently pushing against his ischium, I created a *very subtle* wave of movement through the dog's bones while his muscles remained relaxed. The muscles had the novel experience of staying soft as they "went along for the ride" on the bones. This can relieve sore, tight muscles.

But I was after more than temporary muscular relief. I wanted Nicky's brain to change. Because the skeletal support produced a unique and pleasurable sensation, I knew that the dog's brain would pay attention to it. And attentive brains can learn to recreate movements that feel good. In order to do that, Nicky's brain would have to release the *habit* of chronically contracting muscles. This change in the brain can create long-lasting improvements in the dog's movement and well-being. *Simply put, my skeletal support created a learning experience for the dog. It reminded Nicky that his movement could be easy and comfortable if he didn't habitually tense his muscles.*

Debono Moves promotes relaxation and freer movement throughout the dog's entire body.

---

[15] We have ischia too. They are the bones that you sit on, and are referred to as "sit bones," "seat bones," and "sitz bones" in humans. Please refer to Human Exercise #3, *Easier Sitting,* in Chapter Eight, to learn how you can sit more comfortably on your ischia!

I continued working with Nicky, supporting and moving various parts of his body. He stayed relaxed throughout, even as I gently turned him onto his right side. Since *Debono Moves* induces changes in a dog's *overall state*, Nicky had already released much of the restrictions on his left side before I turned him. I only needed a few minutes to let Nicky experience how comfortable and easy movement on his left side could feel too.

Vicki and I then encouraged the little guy to stand up. I gently moved his pelvis and ribcage, noting how free they now felt. I hoped that Nicky's brain would recognize that moving his pelvis and ribcage made it easier to turn his neck, reducing its stress and strain[16].

As Vicki and I began to walk, Nicky followed us. We were happy to see that the dog's head was held at a more natural angle, and he began turning it to look around. It was a lovely improvement from just an hour ago. But while the *Debono Moves* session could improve Nicky's chances of a complete recovery from his neck injury, Vicki would still need to keep her little dynamo quiet, and to follow-up with her veterinarian. I'm happy to say that Nicky recovered fully and, at over 18 years of age, he is still an active and happy dog!

Learning for Life

I looked on in surprise as the two women claimed their space on the carpeted floor and began moving slowly and mindfully along with the class of new *Feldenkrais Method*® students. These graceful, flexible women were long-time *Feldenkrais*® teachers. What were they doing on the floor? Didn't they already know how to move well?

---

[16] You can experience this increased neck mobility yourself with Human Exercise #5, *Stirring the Soup*, in Chapter Eight.

Boy, did I have a lot to learn! Over time I realized that the two teachers moved so elegantly in their golden years *because* they continued to get on the floor and learn. These women realized that health requires the ability to recover from setbacks, both minor and major ones. It means reminding your nervous system what comfort and ease feel like after a long, tiring day spent cramped in a car or in front of a computer. It means being able to rediscover the joy of movement after surgery to repair a fractured femur. Being healthy means continuing to learn and improve, day after day, year after year. It means caring about the *quality* of your life right now, with an eye towards your future.[17]

The same is true for dogs. While I've helped many canines make significant improvements after just one or two *Debono Moves* sessions, most dogs require several sessions to change long-standing habits and to address new challenges that may crop up. And most importantly, dogs can *continually* improve their well-being when *Debono Moves* is shared with them throughout their lifetimes. That's why I focus on teaching people how to use *Debono Moves* with their animal companions. It's an approach best used as a *way of life* that nurtures connection, awareness and enhanced well-being for dogs and their humans.

Human Exercise #5: Stirring the Soup

Benefits: Many people habitually slump, which can wreak havoc on one's body over time. This exercise can counter that tendency by helping you sit upright effortlessly. It can also improve the mobility of your ribcage, back and pelvis. As we've seen with Nicky, improving the movement

---

[17] In addition to the exercises that accompany this book, we offer educational products at www.DebonoMoves.com/Products. Availing yourself of as many different opportunities to learn will give your brain and body the greatest benefit.

of those areas can enhance the flexibility and comfort of the neck and shoulders.

Plus, when you have elegant posture, you look – and feel – years younger!

Stirring the Soup will also help you do *Ribcage Circles* with your dog more easily and effectively, helping your dog feel better too.

Listen to the audio recording of this exercise by going to www.debonomoves.com/dog-book and typing in the password *free*.

The exercise is printed and illustrated in Chapter Eight.

Ribcage Circles

Benefits may include:

- Increases flexibility and reduces strain on neck and back.

- Promotes healthier, more balanced movement.

- Relaxing and bonding for dog and human.

- Provides all these same benefits for you too.

View a video of Mary teaching *Ribcage Circles* by going to www.debonomoves.com/dog-book and typing in the password *free*.

> **It is important that you do Human Exercise #5, *Stirring the Soup*, before you do this move with your dog.**

Positions: *Ribcage Circles* can be done with your dog sitting, lying on her side, lying like a sphinx or standing up. I explain how to work with your dog in each position.

Let's start with sitting. We'll do this first part without your dog. If you're comfortable sitting on the floor, do the exercise there. You can put your legs out in front of you or sit cross-legged. Better yet, try it both ways and choose the more comfortable option. If you're happier in a chair, find one with a flat seat, like a kitchen chair.

Do Human Exercise #5, *Stirring the Soup.* Pay particular attention to the part of the exercise where you shift your weight around in a circle. Do that movement a few times in each direction, but this time lightly place your hands on your lower ribs. Can you feel your ribcage moving as you shift your pelvis in a circle? Take your hands off your ribs. Continue circling, but now *hold your hands softly in front of you.* Let your movement feel light and easy. If you're sitting on the floor, do you move differently than when you are in a chair?

Practice with your dog. Call your dog over to you. If you are sitting on the floor, ask your dog to sit and stay, and then move so that you are sitting behind your dog. If you prefer to be in a chair, ask your dog to sit on the couch or some other surface that allows you to sit in a chair across from her. You will be sitting very close to your dog. If possible, you and your dog will be facing in the same direction.

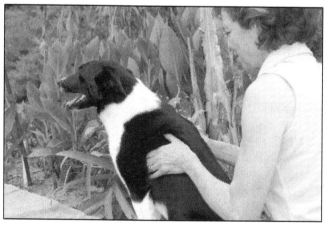

With my hands held lightly on Maggie's ribcage, I slowly move my pelvis in a circle. This induces a subtle circular movement in the dog's ribcage, which can help keep her back, shoulders and neck limber.

Lightly place your hands on either side of your dog's ribcage. Take a moment to simply breathe with your dog in this position. Then slowly shift your weight around in a circle, like you did in *Stirring the Soup*. Since your hands connect your dog's body to you, your dog's ribcage will start to move very, very lightly in a circle. *This is a small, subtle movement.* If you feel resistance, reduce your pressure. The movement should feel delicate and easy for both you and your dog.

Do the movement a few times in each direction. Notice if there are places where the movement seems less free than other places. Do you and your dog have less-easy spots in the same places on the circle? If so, does improving *your* movement help your dog improve as well?

Do several circles in each direction.

Ask your dog to lie on her chest, like a sphinx.

You can follow the sitting directions above for the sphinx position. Your dog has more of her body contacting the surface she is resting on.

Does that change how her ribcage moves? What else is different for you and your dog?

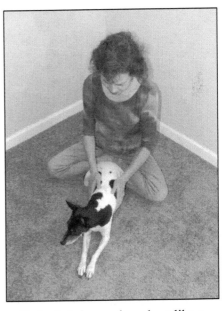

Ruby is lying on her chest like a sphinx.

Ask your dog to lie flat on her side. Again, position yourself so that you are sitting very close to your dog. Place both hands on one side of your dog's ribcage, on the side that is facing up. If your dog is lying on her right side, both your hands will rest lightly on her left side.

Shift your weight around in slow, easy circles. Can you feel your dog's ribcage move as you move? Keep your hands soft and light. Are you breathing? Is your dog breathing in a relaxed way? Do several circles in each direction. Then ask your dog to lie on her other side and explore the movements on that side. Does one side move more easily than the other?

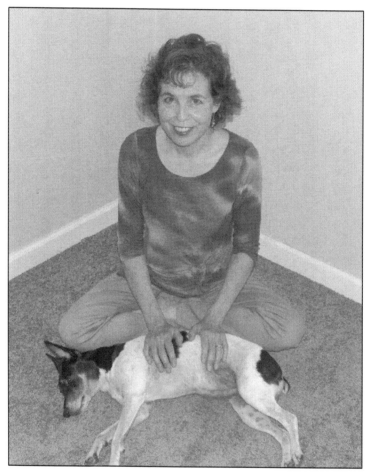

As I move my pelvis in slow, easy circles, Ruby's ribcage moves too.

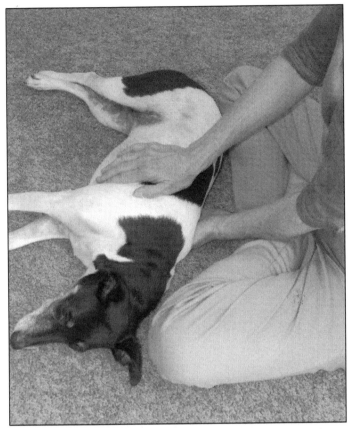

You can also do *Ribcage Circles* with one hand
on each side.

Your dog will be standing up. If your dog is standing
on the floor, you can kneel next to her. Alternately, you can
carefully place your dog on a wall or table and stand next to
her. Make sure that whatever surface you choose is not
slippery for your dog. Please do the following explorations
before calling your dog over.

If you plan to kneel next to your dog, take off your shoes
and kneel on a comfortable surface, such as a carpet, folded

towel or a kneeling pad that gardeners use. If you stand, wear flat shoes or bare feet.

Whether kneeling or standing, slowly shift your pelvis in a circle. How does it feel to shift your weight when you are kneeling or standing? Are some parts of the circle easier than others? You may have to make the circles smaller to make them smooth and light. Do a few easy circles in each direction.

Place your hands on your lower ribs and do a few more circles. Feel the movement in your ribcage. Now lightly hold your hands out in front of you and circle your pelvis.

When you feel ready, invite your dog over and encourage her to stand. Face the same direction your dog is facing.

*Please note that leaning your body or putting your arm over the back of a dog can be threatening to some canines. I recommend that you **not** do this with dogs who are timid, aggressive, unfamiliar to you, or in any way uncomfortable. Only do what is pleasant and safe for you and your dog.*

Put the arm that is next to your dog over her back so that your hand softly contacts your dog's ribs. Place your other hand on the side of her ribcage that is closest to you.

Breathe with her for a minute or so, then imagine moving your pelvis in a circle. After a few imaginary circles, actually shift your pelvis in slow, lazy circles.

Make sure that you are not leaning on your dog. Keep your arms light and relaxed all the way to your fingertips. Do a few circles in each direction. Gradually bring the circles to a stop. Pause for a moment before you remove your hands. Praise and thank your dog.

Move to your dog's other side or ask your dog to turn around. Put a hand on each side of her ribcage again. Does this side feel different to you? It's possible that it'll be easier to put one arm over your dog's back compared to the other. Notice if that is true for you. Can you modify the position so that it's comfortable for you? You can face the opposite direction so that your other arm goes over your dog's back.

Mary's Tip:

Keep in mind that your intent is to create a calming, enjoyable and educational experience for you and your dog. *Slower, lighter* movements will reap the most benefit.

Novelty and variation stimulate the brain to learn. The more positions (i.e., sitting, sphinx, lying flat and standing) your dog can *comfortably* be in while you do a *Debono Move*, the greater the possibility of improvement.

Shoulder and Ribcage Circles

View a video of Mary teaching *Shoulder and Ribcage Circles* by going to www.debonomoves.com/dog-book and typing in the password *free.*

Benefits may include:

- Increases flexibility and reduces strain on neck, forelegs and back.
- Novel movements stimulate the brain to discover easier, healthier movement.
- Helps improve your coordination and body awareness too.

Practice with a human friend first. It can be helpful to practice *Shoulder and Ribcage Circles* with a human friend first. Ask your friend to lie on her side with her knees comfortably drawn up. Place a small pillow under her head to support her neck. Place one hand on your friend's shoulder blade and the other on the side of her ribcage. Then follow the instructions below. Trade places so that you both give and receive *Shoulder and Ribcage Circles*. Not only will this give you an idea of what your dog feels, but your friend's feedback can help improve your technique.

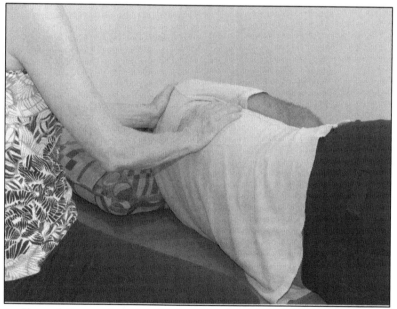

I'm subtly moving Gary's shoulder blade in clockwise circles and his ribcage in counterclockwise circles.

Position: Dog is lying flat on his side.

Practice with your dog. For this exercise, your dog should be lying on his side. Position yourself so that you are sitting behind him, facing his back. If it's comfortable for you, sit on the floor, either cross-legged or with your legs spread apart. Alternately, you can also ask your dog to lie down on your sofa or bed, and you can either pull up a chair or sit next to him.

While sitting comfortably upright, put one hand on your dog's shoulder and the other on his ribcage. Just relax in this position and breathe. After a minute or so, begin to make light, **counterclockwise** circles with the hand that is on your dog's shoulder. Your hand stays in contact with your dog. While your pressure should be light, you are doing more than simply moving the skin around. You should feel a *very subtle* movement of your dog's shoulder blade. Make several counterclockwise circles and then pause. Keep your hand on your dog's shoulder.

With the hand that is on your dog's ribcage, make light **clockwise** circles. Again, this is a very subtle movement. Keep it light. Don't use force. Pause after several circles.

Simultaneously do counterclockwise circles with the hand on your dog's shoulder hand and clockwise circles with the hand on the ribcage. Notice how this movement affects *your* upper back and shoulders. Make the circles light and easy. It can be helpful to visualize a clock under each hand. In addition to going in opposite directions, your hands should be at opposite "hours" on the clocks.

After several movements, reverse the direction of your circles so that you are making clockwise circles with your dog's shoulder and counterclockwise circles with his ribcage. Is this easier or more challenging for you?

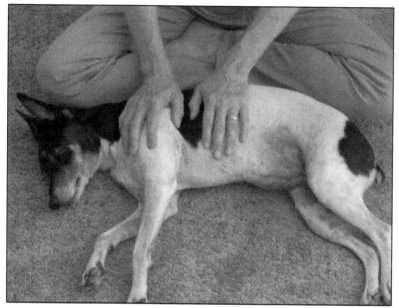

My right hand moves in slow circles on Ruby's shoulder while my left hand moves her ribcage in circles in the opposite direction. My contact is light and gentle at all times.

When practicing with a human friend, notice how it feels if you move the shoulder and ribs in the same direction (i.e., both clockwise or both counterclockwise) versus making them in opposing directions. Most people prefer the opposing directions. In addition, opposing circles usually bring about the greatest improvement in coordination and flexibility in both the person practicing the move and the individual receiving it.

Human Exercise #6: Turning Toward a Supple Spine

Benefits: This exercise can help you move more parts of your spine, which helps you turn more easily. It can also improve the movement and comfort of your neck, back and hips.

Listen to the audio recording of this exercise by going to www.debonomoves.com/dog-book and typing in the password *free*.

The exercise is printed and illustrated in Chapter Eight.

Key Points of Chapter Four

- Rhythmic movements (such as *Rhythm Circles*) can stimulate relaxation and healing.

- Using your fingertips to lift and support soft tissue can provide relief to sore, tight muscles.

- As you gently touch your dog, imagine sending out healing vibrations that spread like ripples in a pond.

- Enhancing the movement of the ribcage can reduce strain in the neck.

- Novel movements help the brain discover easier, healthier movement options.

- The more variations of a move (sitting, sphinx, lying, and standing) you and your dog comfortably explore, the greater the possibility of improvement.

- Supporting a dog's skeleton can free up the muscles. And change the brain.

- *Debono Moves* can promote a change in the dog's *overall state*, resulting in a calmer mind and freer movement.

- Dogs and humans can continue to learn and improve over their lifetimes.

- Use *Debono Moves* to create a calming, enjoyable experience for you and your dog.
- *Debono Moves* is best used as a *way of life* that nurtures connection, awareness and enhanced well-being for dogs and their people.

Chapter Five: What Do Torn Knee Ligaments, Arthritis, and Habits Have in Common?

Do you slump when you're watching TV or sitting in front of a computer? Do you react to stress by tensing your shoulders? Do you stand on one leg more than the other? These, and other less visible habits, may cause stiff joints and achy muscles.

And, you guessed it, dogs can have bad habits too! Below, you'll find the stories of two dogs who inadvertently caused their own lameness. The first dog, Sonny, is a yellow Lab who had surgery to repair a torn knee ligament. The second dog, Jackson, is an Airedale who was diagnosed with arthritis. Both dogs stopped limping when I helped them release their inefficient habits and replace them with body confidence.

The exercises in this chapter can help you identify if you and your dog have habits that are interfering with comfort and well-being. Then I'll take you through some steps to release those inefficient patterns and replace them with movements that increase vitality and well-being.

Sonny Heals His Torn Knee Ligament

The sound of barking dogs greeted me as I strode up the slate steps. A small woman with short, black curly hair and a smile in her voice called out, "Come on in!" as she wrangled the canines away from the door. There were three of them – a gigantic Tibetan Mastiff, a yellow Labrador Retriever and a chocolate Lab. I knew immediately who I was there to see; the yellow Lab who was enthusiastically wagging his tail while balancing on three legs.

Sonny, this exuberant five-year-old Lab, had torn a ligament in his right knee. He underwent surgery to repair his cranial cruciate ligament (oftentimes referred to as the anterior cruciate ligament or "ACL")[18]. The surgery went well and Sonny was expected to return to full activity following a period of rest and rehabilitation. However, it was now ten months since the surgery and Sonny was still limping. His surgeon was at a loss to explain why.

Even when Sonny put his right hind foot on the ground, it was clear that he carried more of his weight on his left hind leg. And when Sonny walked, he had a distinct limp. The dog's body showed the tell-tale signs of this asymmetrical balancing act: his back was constantly tense, the muscles of his right hind leg had atrophied and the muscles of his left hind leg were taut. Sonny's tight shoulders also indicated the extra work his front legs were doing.

Dogs can limp out of habit.

Since the veterinary surgeon could find no reason for the dog's continual limp, it was possible that Sonny's habit of protecting his injured, painful leg had become so ingrained that he had forgotten what it was like *not* to limp. He had spent months guarding against pain, first from the injury and then from the surgery. In doing so, Sonny had lost the supple, confident use of his body. His continued limping put a constant strain on his opposite hind leg, leaving him pre-disposed to tearing *that* CCL. We certainly wanted to avoid that!

My job was to help Sonny feel that moving freely was safer and more comfortable than limping. To do this, I tapped into the same bodily wisdom – the nervous system – that created the limp in the first place. After all, limping is an

---

[18] While many people use the term "ACL" when speaking about their dogs, it is more accurately referred to as the *cranial cruciate ligament* or "CCL" in dogs.

intelligent response to pain, protecting the injured area and helping to reduce discomfort. The drawback only comes when the limp has outlived its usefulness, and the imbalance creates strain and the potential for further damage. Since the limp was now an impediment, it was clearly time for the Labrador to let it go.

It's a bad idea to force a dog to stand on the leg he is protecting.

Some people force the dog to stand on the surgically-repaired leg by holding up the opposite leg or rocking the dog's weight over to the injured side. But without the proper preparation, the dog's nervous system would flag that as unsafe and develop additional compensations, such as further tightening of the back. In contrast, gentle, safe and pleasurable movements do not elicit the body's defenses. Since the nervous system is hard-wired to recreate pleasurable sensations, comfortable movements are more likely to influence the dog's functioning. The dog gains confidence and the improvement is more likely to "stick."

Positive reinforcement can help calm an excited or distracted dog.

I went over to Sonny's dog bed and encouraged him to lie down. Sonny did as he was asked, but quickly popped up again. We repeated this a few times. Tail constantly wagging, Sonny was just too excited to lie down while there was a new person in his home! It is certainly possible for me to work with dogs while they are standing up (I do it with horses all the time), but lying down would allow Sonny's muscles to relax, giving me more opportunities to move his back and legs, and generally allow for quicker results.

It's been my experience that most dogs will begin to settle down and enjoy the session once they feel that *my hands are offering them a way out of their usual discomfort.* The key is to get their attention in such a way that they *can* experience this change.

There are many ways to approach this. Since Sonny knew the verbal cue, "Down," I started there. Each time Sonny responded to my request by lying down on his bed, he received a small piece of dog biscuit. Since he wanted to immediately stand up and play, I *very gradually* increased the time between Sonny's correct response (lying down) and his reward (the treat). Subtlety and patience are essential. If you increase the interval between the cue and treat too much, too soon, the dog will just give up and leave. If, on the other hand, you keep handing over treats non-stop, the dog doesn't learn how to stay in position, and it would be difficult to get anything accomplished.

Each time Sonny lay down, I used my hands to gently lift and support the muscles along his back. I worked down one side of his spine and up the other. My movements were light, slow and rhythmic. Sonny soon began to relax.

Sonny learned that movement could be balanced and comfortable.

Little by little, Sonny became more focused on what I was doing and we relied on the treats less and less. The lifting motion helped relieve the tension in those overworked back muscles. Even more importantly, Sonny experienced that movement in his back was *possible* and *comfortable.*

This is an important step in creating change – letting the animal experience that *it's possible to feel differently.* This helps break the vicious cycle of habits and allows change to be not only *possible*, but an easier and more comfortable option.

After slowly outlining Sonny's spine on both sides, I placed my hands on the fullness of his ribcage and I delicately slid his ribcage in various directions. This helped to relieve the strain in his shoulders and neck. I also worked with Sonny's sternum and individual ribs, reminding him that these parts could move. I supported the muscles along Sonny's shoulders, which elicited great, deep breaths of apparent appreciation. At this point, Sonny had stopped thinking about getting up to play or investigate any noises.

I supported and guided Sonny's body, letting him feel how his different parts could move easily and comfortably. I always kept the movements safe and easy, continually checking the dog for any signs of stress. I noted the depth and rate of his breathing, the look in his eyes, and the set of his ears and tail. To reduce the chance of anxiety, I worked with his non-injured side first. I alternated between moving the left hind leg, then the right hind leg, so Sonny could experience how the movement of both hind legs felt similarly safe and comfortable. As we ended that first session, Sonny was more comfortable and relaxed in his body, although the limp was still present.

Non-habitual movements reinforced the Labrador's progress.

I returned several more times to work with this lovely dog. Since the brain is stimulated by novelty and variation, I used non-habitual movements in various ways to reinforce Sonny's learning. As with Rocky, I used a small hardcover book under his paws *("Artificial Floor")* to help Sonny "stand" on first his left hind leg, then his right, all while he was safely and comfortably lying down. This allowed him to experience "standing" with a relaxed back. I imagine that it had been quite a long time since his nervous system associated standing with a supple back.

The dog's whole body now moved in a healthy, coordinated way.

Now that he was prepared, it was important that Sonny learn how to keep his back flexible as he *actually* stood and moved. If he did not, his tight back would interfere with his freedom of movement and could set him up for further orthopedic problems down the road. To show Sonny how his back could remain supple, I asked the yellow Lab to stand, and I lightly moved his hips, pelvis, spine and ribs. I then gently shifted his weight in a circle, allowing him to feel how he could now bear weight comfortably on all four limbs, including his surgically-repaired right hind leg. This was very different than forcing the Labrador to stand on the leg he was favoring. The circles gave Sonny the experience of shifting his weight *safely and effortlessly* from leg to leg, which allowed him to gradually give up the habit of protecting his right hind leg. [19]

Afterward, I encouraged Sonny to walk, and I was happy to notice how much freer he looked. *Now that Sonny had improved his coordination, the different parts of his body worked together to share the effort of moving.* Happily, Sonny's limp disappeared after several *Debono Moves* sessions. This exuberant Labrador had regained confidence in his body and could once again run and play with joy.

---

[19] To understand what it means to shift a dog's weight in a circle, try this exercise. As with all the exercises, do not proceed if there is any discomfort. Find a carpeted area and go on all fours. Your weight will be on your hands and knees. If it's difficult to put your palms on the ground, place your fists on the ground and keep your wrists straight. Notice how your weight is distributed over your four limbs. Shift your body so that you take more weight onto your left hand. Keep the weight there for only a second or so, and then shift your weight onto your left knee, then your right knee and then your right hand. You just shifted your weight in a circle.

Now do it again, noticing what parts of your body move to accommodate your weight shift. Can you feel your torso, pelvis and head responding? Can you make the movements lighter and faster, so that you reduce the pressure on each of your four limbs? Remember that the lighter your movements are, the more you will feel. The more you feel, the more you can improve. Explore how easily you can shift your weight from limb to limb in a circle. Does moving other parts of your body help you shift your weight effortlessly? Change the direction of your circles and notice any differences.

Jackson Stops Arthritis in Its Tracks

Dark-haired and impeccably dressed, Mary Jane entered through the glass door of my office with her Airedale, Jackson, limping along by her side. Although his left front leg was obviously bothering him, the black-and-tan dog didn't let it affect his attitude. Body wiggling, he greeted me as if I were a long-lost friend. As I squatted down beside her dog, Mary Jane explained that a veterinarian's examination and X-rays had shown that her dog had arthritis in his left carpus, the area similar to our wrist.

Even young dogs can be diagnosed with arthritis.

Mary Jane had not expected such a diagnosis. It would be one thing if her dog were geriatric, or even mature. But Jackson was only three years old! How could he have arthritis? She was dismayed to hear the words *"degenerative changes"* and *"arthritis"* spoken about her young dog. They were such hopeless words. Words that suggested a future filled with increasing pain, stiffness and reduced mobility. Mary Jane was concerned how arthritis would affect Jackson's quality of life now and in the future, and she wondered if there was a way to change the course of her beloved dog's condition. So when a friend suggested that *Debono Moves* could be helpful, Mary Jane didn't hesitate to contact me.

As I stroked the handsome Airedale, I too wondered why such a young dog would develop arthritis. And then I set to work to find the answer.

With Jackson standing quietly, I delicately shifted his weight in different directions. These explorations allowed me to sense how Jackson *habitually* carried his weight before the pain of arthritis caused him to modify his movement.

What I discovered was that Jackson had a habit of bearing more weight on his left front leg. Yes, the leg that had developed painful arthritis. Sure, he took his weight off that leg now that it hurt so badly; but when I asked him to shift his weight in different directions, he returned time and again to loading that limb more than the others. The asymmetrical development of some of his muscles also pointed to this left foreleg bias.[20]

Over time, unbalanced movement can cause wear and tear damage.

You may wonder why Jackson was using his body asymmetrically. It is possible that at some earlier time the Airedale sustained an injury, even a minor one, on his right side. He may have compensated for the discomfort by slightly favoring his right side, which caused him to carry more weight on his left front limb. Since that strategy helped him feel better, he continued it, even long after it was helpful. Over time it became a habit and felt normal to the dog. But uneven

---

[20] To accurately learn how Jackson organized his weight, my movements had to be very light and precise. Anyone can shift a dog's weight from side-to-side by pushing on the dog, but in order to determine which direction was easier for Jackson to shift to, my touch had to be barely perceptible.

Think about it this way. Let's say you are carrying a heavy box of books. A butterfly lands on the box, but you cannot tell when it flies off. Because you are using a lot of effort to carry the box, your nervous system cannot discriminate when such a small difference – the weight of a butterfly – is added or removed.

Now let's pretend you are holding a feather lightly between your thumb and forefinger. A butterfly lands on the feather. You can immediately feel the increased weight in your hand. A decrease in weight will tell you that the butterfly has taken flight.

It's the same when we are touching our dogs. When we use greater effort, our bodies cannot discriminate between subtle differences in sensation. But when we use a minimum amount of pressure, we are able to discern even small differences in ease of movement. These small but important differences are what we are looking for.

And it's true for the dog as well. If you use a very small amount of pressure, the canine's nervous system can recognize, and learn from, the subtle differences. If you use a greater amount of force, all the dog feels is that he is being pushed to the side.

limb loading, however subtle, can cause increased strain on joints and muscles. If it goes on long enough, injury can occur.[21]

Whatever the cause of his asymmetry, I knew that I had something important to teach Jackson. While *Debono Moves* resembles gentle bodywork, it is actually an educational approach. *Debono Moves* could help Jackson learn to move in a way that wouldn't overstress his left front wrist, or any other any area.

Releasing tense muscles enhances relaxa-tion, develops trust and helps the dog move efficiently and comfortably.

With Jackson now lying quietly on a royal blue dog mat, I supported his tense muscles that were fatigued from compensating for his painful leg. This elicited deep, audible breaths from the Airedale. *Helping your dog release sore, tense muscles enhances relaxation, develops trust, and allows the dog's nervous system to focus on learning.*

I then used my hands to guide different parts of his body through gentle, novel movements, which can help stimulate the creation of new neural connections. Such neural activity meant that the Airedale would be less likely to be stuck in his habitual, unbalanced way of moving, but instead have healthier movement options.

The less pressure you use with your dog, the more you and your dog can feel.

After working with the dog for about 40 minutes, I began exploring the movements of his front leg joints. I was very careful to make only light, delicate movements that were barely more than a thought. Since *Debono Moves* works by engaging the dog's brain, small gentle movements are usually

---

[21] See "When Good Habits Go Bad," in this chapter, to learn more about the role of habits.

best. *Keep in mind that the less pressure you use, the more you and your dog will feel. The more one feels, the more one can improve.*

In addition, these small movements did not invoke a protective response from the dog. In contrast, large, potentially-uncomfortable manipulations can create muscular "armoring" around the joint, which further limits its movement. Anxiety about being hurt also prevents the dog from learning a healthier way to move.

I associated Jackson's new movement possibilities with comfort and ease.

And even though Jackson's right wrist *could* have easily and safely been taken through a greater range of motion, I only moved it the *same amount* that his left wrist could easily move. This provided Jackson with an equal sense of easy mobility in *both* legs. *I wanted Jackson to feel the possibilities of movement in his left leg by associating them with comfort and pleasure.* By alternatively moving the dog's left and right wrists, I helped strengthen this association.[22]

Again, the dog was creating new neural pathways between his brain and his left leg. Hopefully, it would enable him to use his leg in an easier, more functional way. The Airedale, still lying on his side, remained relaxed and comfortable throughout the session.

While it was wonderful to see how good Jackson felt while he was lying down, it was time for him to experience that he could now *walk* better too. So after asking the young dog to stand up, I gently shifted his weight in a smooth, even circle. This exercise let the Airedale feel how he could use all four of his limbs in a more balanced way, something he was not able to do when he limped into my office. To further

---

[22] You may have noticed that I don't use the terms "good leg" and "bad leg" in referring to Jackson's limbs. Describing your dog, or yourself, in those terms can leave a lasting imprint of limitation and preclude full healing.

enhance Jackson's body awareness, I put my hands on various parts of his body as Mary Jane asked her dog to walk around my office.

Jackson left the office that day without a limp. He was, according to Mary Jane, "a new dog." And while the reader may be left wondering how one *Debono Moves* session could possibly cure arthritis, I have an explanation. Jackson's arthritis *wasn't* cured. If a radiograph was taken immediately following the session, it would look the same as it did before the session. Based on X-rays alone, it would appear as if the session had done nothing helpful at all.

For long-lasting improvement, I addressed the *cause* of the Airedale's arthritis.

What *Debono Moves* did was help the Airedale release the neuromuscular tension that caused much of his acute soreness and stiffness. And even more importantly, Jackson discovered how to move in a way that reduced the stress on his joints and muscles. That is why giving a dog pain-relieving medication, *without resolving the underlying issue that is causing the arthritis,* simply masks the pain.

It doesn't stop the cycle of excessive wear and tear. And although he received sessions later in his life for minor sports injuries, the arthritis in his left foreleg stopped being a problem for Jackson. As a matter of fact, I took to calling him *Action Jackson* due to his high energy and athletic prowess!

It was fortunate that Jackson's carpal arthritis was diagnosed at an early stage, before the arthritis caused significant deterioration of his carpal joints. Unfortunately, that is often not the case. Since many dogs develop arthritis slowly, they gradually become accustomed to the stiffness and discomfort. These dogs often do not limp or otherwise reveal their problem until the arthritis becomes more advanced.

Jackson's limp and Mary Jane's quick action allowed her dog to make a full and speedy recovery.[23]

Scanning Your Dog's Body

Benefits may include:

- Enhances your dog's body awareness.

- Accustoms your dog to being gently and comfortably handled.

- May alert you to the first signs of injury or illness so you can seek immediate veterinary care.

- Allows you to recognize if your dog moves in a balanced way.

At the start of each human exercise that accompanies this book, I ask you to check in with yourself before you begin to move. For example, I suggest that you compare your right and left sides, noticing if one side feels tighter, longer or wider. Even though this "body scan" is done while standing still, it can tell you a lot about how you move. It also helps direct your attention to different parts of yourself, shining a light on areas that you may have tuned out.

---

[23] It is not uncommon for canine athletes to develop carpal arthritis, but you can minimize the chance of your dog developing it. These complex joints, which act as shock absorbers, do not have a lot of muscular support. This makes them prone to repetitive injury, especially if a dog habitually bears weight unevenly. You may find the exercises in this book helpful in improving your dog's movement and balance. Additionally, if you haven't already had your young pup's dewclaws removed, you may want to consider keeping them. It is likely that the dewclaws reduce the torque that is applied to the dog's front legs, especially when turning at the canter and gallop. Less torque equals less wear and tear damage to the carpus. This is especially important for dogs that participate in agility, flyball and other canine sports that require turning at speed. See *Do the Dew(claws)?* written by M. Christine Zink, DVM, PhD, DACVSMR; www.caninesports.com.

In much the same way, you can learn about your dog by doing an introductory *Debono Moves* **Body Scan** with your canine companion. Your dog can also benefit from the enhanced body awareness your exploration provides.

Position: A *Body Scan* can be done with your dog standing, sitting and lying down. Skip any position that is uncomfortable for you or your dog.

Begin by watching your dog as he moves freely around your house or yard. Is he favoring a part of his body? Please contact your dog's veterinarian if you suspect pain or movement limitations.

Standing

With your dog standing in a relaxed way, slowly slide your hands up your dog's hind legs to feel his muscles. Is one leg more developed than the other? If so, it may indicate that your dog is using that leg more than its mate. Run your hands up the front legs.

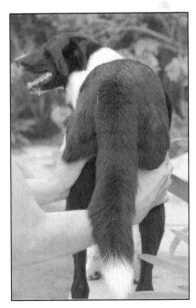

Do you notice any differences? Is one shoulder area more developed than the other?

Gently and slowly slide your hands from the base of his skull to the tip of his tail. Does your dog's back quiver when it's touched? Become familiar with your dog's muscle tone throughout his body.

I compare the size and tone in the muscles of Maggie's hind legs.

95

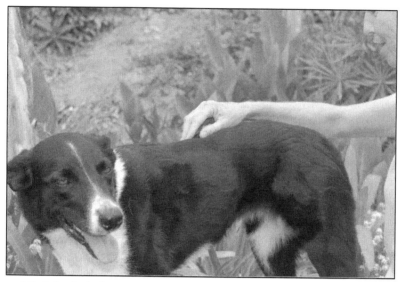

I lightly feel along Maggie's back, noting if there are any areas of tension.

Sitting

Does your dog sit squarely or does he lean on one hip? Some dogs, especially puppies, sit off to the side. In mature dogs, this may indicate a problem. Notice if he always sits on the same hip. Inform your veterinarian if your dog habitually sits crooked.

Lying Down

With your dog lying on his side, examine his paws. Do his nails wear evenly? How do his paw pads feel and look? Is the wear even? Does he allow you to check in between his toes?

Feel the top-lying front and hind leg muscles, then have your dog gently roll onto his other side and repeat the inspection. Do you notice a difference in the development of your dog's leg muscles?

Gently run your hands from your dog's head to tail, including his ribcage and abdomen. Use a light, listening contact. Scanning your dog on a regular basis will alert you to potential problems that require a vet's attention.

Human Exercise #7: Hip and Shoulder Circles

Benefits: This exercise can help you enjoy freer movement in your pelvis and shoulders, while it facilitates more balanced, coordinated movement throughout your whole body.

It can also improve your ability to do *Hip and Shoulder Circles* with your dog so you can help your canine companion move more freely too!

Listen to the audio recording of this exercise by going to www.debonomoves.com/dog-book and typing in the password *free*.

The exercise is printed and illustrated in Chapter Eight.

Hip and Shoulder Circles

View a video of Mary teaching *Hip and Shoulder Circles* by going to www.debonomoves.com/dog-book and typing in the password *free*.

Benefits may include:

- Helps relieve stress around shoulders and hips.

- Novel movements stimulate the brain to discover easier, healthier movement.

- Reminds your dog how to move in a more balanced way.

- Enhances your coordination and improves *your* shoulder movement too.

Practice with a human friend first. It can be helpful to practice *Hip and Shoulder Circles* with a human friend before you do it with your dog. Ask your friend to lie on her side with her knees comfortably drawn up. Place a small pillow under her head to support her neck. Place one hand on your friend's shoulder blade and the other on her pelvis ("hip bone"), and then follow the instructions below. Trade places so that you both give and receive *Hip and Shoulder Circles.* Not only will this give you an idea of what your dog feels, but your friend's feedback can help improve your technique.

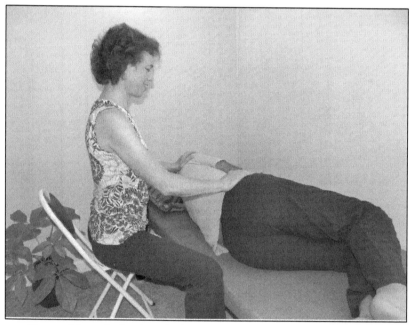

I'm making clockwise circles with Gary's shoulder blade and counterclockwise circles with his pelvis ("hip bone").

Position: Dog is lying flat on her side.

Practice with your dog. For this exercise, your dog should be lying on her side. Position yourself so that you are sitting behind her, facing her back. If it's comfortable for you, sit on the floor, either cross-legged or with your legs spread apart. Alternately, you can ask your dog to lie down on your sofa or bed, and you can either pull up a chair or sit next to her.

While sitting comfortably upright, put one hand on your dog's shoulder and the other on her hip. Just relax in this position and breathe. After a minute or so, begin to make light, **clockwise** circles with the hand that is on your dog's shoulder. Your hand stays in contact with your dog. While your pressure should be light, you are doing more than simply moving the skin around. You should feel a *very subtle* movement of your dog's shoulder blade. Make several clockwise circles and then pause. Keep your hand on your dog's shoulder.

With the hand that is on your dog's hip, make light **counterclockwise** circles. Again, this is a very subtle movement. You may notice your dog's leg moving a tiny bit. Keep it light. Don't use force. Pause after several circles.

Simultaneously do clockwise circles with the hand on your dog's shoulder hand and counterclockwise circles with the hand on her hip. Notice how this movement affects *your* upper back and shoulders. Make the circles light and easy. It can be helpful to visualize a clock under each hand. In addition to going in opposite directions, your hands should be at opposite "hours" on the clocks.

When practicing with a human friend, notice how it feels if you make the circles in the same direction versus making them in opposing directions. Most people prefer opposing circles. In addition, opposing circles usually bring about the greatest improvement in coordination and flexibility in both the person practicing the move and the individual receiving it.

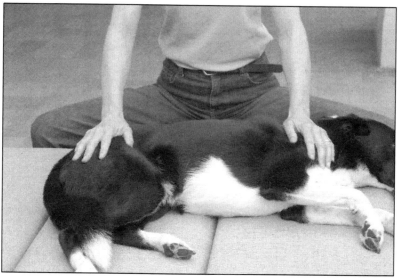

Hip and Shoulder Circles. Note that Maggie is lying on a chaise while I sit comfortably on a stool behind her.

Mary's Tip:

To understand how little pressure is needed or desired for *Debono Moves*, use only one-tenth of the pressure that you think you should use. That means you reduce your effort by 90%. If you believe that amount of pressure couldn't possibly do anything useful, remember this: *the less pressure you use, the more high-quality sensory information you give your dog.* Less effort equals more improvement!

When Good Habits Go Bad

Have you ever stubbed your toe really hard? If you did, you probably limped to protect your aching foot. The throbbing from a stubbed toe usually resolves fairly quickly and it's likely that you went back to walking without a limp in no time. But if you suffered an injury that took longer to heal, things may not be that simple. You probably adopted long-term ways of holding and moving your body to compensate for your injury.

Time passes and your injury heals, so you resume your usual activities. You take your dog on long hikes, go running and work out. Everything seems fine. But some months or even years later, trouble starts. You notice an annoying crick in your neck. Or your back feels sore and stiff. Or maybe your knee or hip starts to bother you. Because you didn't suffer a recent injury, you chalk up these aches and pains to aging. That's what happens when we get old, right?

Well, no.

Remember those compensations that helped you deal with your injury? You most likely kept a remnant of them long after your injury healed. And not only have they have outlived their usefulness, they are now causing problems of their own. *But since they have become habitual, you don't even notice that you're doing them.*

Why does this happen?

Put simply, the nervous system is responsible for maintaining the body's safety. When an injury occurs, the nervous system registers pain to keep us from using the injured part. We limp to reduce the discomfort, allowing the injured part to rest. It's an effective strategy. Gradually the pain subsides and, in many cases, the limp disappears. Well, almost disappears. In actuality, the nervous system may not entirely let go of the limp. It doesn't want re-injury to occur, so it may retain a trace of the limp. We may unconsciously tense the back muscles more on one side when walking or habitually bear more weight on the unaffected leg. There are as many ways to limp as there are individuals, and it often becomes a habitual and unconscious act.

Such a habit may go unnoticed for years, until problems start developing. Like we saw with Sonny and Jackson, dogs do this too. That is one reason why many dogs end up injuring the opposite cranial cruciate ligament (CCL) months after they tore the first one. After one side has been injured, the dog may never *fully* use that leg, even after the ligament has healed. This causes chronic strain in the opposite hind leg, which can eventually lead to a tear in that CCL. So while some dogs have a genetic predisposition to weak CCLs, for others unequal weight bearing contributes to ligament damage.

You don't have to suffer an injury to develop these kinds of habits. They also develop as a way to deal with everyday stresses and strains. Maybe you've spent years slinging a heavy purse over one shoulder and your body has adjusted to deal with that unbalanced load. Or you spent too much time sitting and developed unhealthy postural habits. Or maybe as a child you hunched up your shoulders every time your parents bickered and that became your habitual response to stress. Eventually these compensations cause you discomfort, so you tense and limit other body parts to cope with the *new* aches and pains. *This vicious cycle tends to age you, fast.*

Fortunately, you can stop this cycle. Just like Sonny and Jackson, you can learn to move freely again. The exercises that accompany this book will help you and your dog release unhealthy habits and embrace easier, more youthful movement.

Taking Off Your Pants Can Keep You Nimble

There's an old saying, *"Everyone puts their pants on one leg at a time."* True enough, but do you always start with the *same* leg when you put on your pants? When you put on a shirt or jacket, do you slip the same arm into the garment first? And how about when you take off your pants or jacket? Which limb do you move first? If you're like many people, you habitually put the same leg into your trousers first. And you slip the same arm into your jacket first. The same holds true for taking them off.

Over a lifetime, we put clothes on and take them off so many times that we don't give it a second thought. The process becomes *habitual.* Habits can be quite useful in saving you time. After all, you wouldn't want to have to think about how to tie your shoes every time you put them on. It's expedient to do some things automatically.

But habits can also limit you mentally and physically. Doing the same things over and over reduces your chances of doing something new and innovative. The neural circuitry associated with habits becomes so deeply ingrained that you no longer seek a better way to do things. Your brain runs on autopilot, diminishing mental and physical flexibility.[24]

In contrast, taking a break from the ordinary can create new neural pathways. It may prevent memory loss as it rewires your brain, awakening your mind and body as more senses are activated. By using your body and mind in non-habitual ways, you can open the door to physical and mental nimbleness.

I've seen this to be true with dogs too. The novel Debono Moves not only help our canine companions move easier, but those with behavioral challenges often act more appropriately too. **Releasing the body from limitations seems to free up the mind.**

It's easy to introduce novelty into your life. The human exercises and canine *Debono Moves* I teach are full of non-

---

[24] See "When Good Habits Go Bad," in this chapter for information on how humans and dogs develop inefficient habits and how they have the potential to cause harm.

habitual movements, so I encourage you to explore them.[25] I've also included some suggestions on how to add variety into your everyday life, but I'm sure you'll come up with a lot more ideas. Just thinking about it will stimulate your brain and create new neural connections!

Novelty and variety can enrich your dog's life as well as your own. Below are some suggestions for non-habitual activities that you can do with your dog:

- Explore new places with your dog and safely meet new canine and human friends.

- Set up an obstacle course that you and your dog can safely navigate. You can walk over poles, step through tires on the ground, and weave around poles. Let your imagination run free as you create a canine-human playground! Both you and your canine companion will benefit from the novel sensory experiences and fun physical challenges.

- Vary the surface you and your dog walk on. Take your dog to diverse places to exercise, such as a sandy beach, a leaf-strewn wooded path, a grassy field and a cement sidewalk. Your dog's brain – and your own – will be stimulated by the different sensations that each surface produces.

- Teach your dog new behaviors.[26]

- Train your dog to walk on your other side.

---

[25] Twelve canine *Debono Moves* are taught in this book. To find out how you can learn more moves for your dog, visit our website at www.DebonoMoves.com/events/canine-workshops. For information on additional human exercises, go to www.DebonoMoves.com/Products.

[26] Improving our skill at dog training using positive reinforcement is good for our brains and for our dogs. I suggest you consult with a qualified professional who teaches positive reinforcement canine training.

- Take different routes on your walks with your dog. If you usually turn right at the end of your driveway, turn left.

- Put on music and play with your dog. Maybe even learn canine freestyle dancing!

- Participate in a canine sport with your dog.

- Learn how to read canine body language. Your dog will thank you.[27]

- Challenge yourself to do even one little thing differently with your dog each day.

Here are more suggestions to add novelty and variety to your life:

- Hold the phone to your other ear.

- Put your clothes on and take them off non-habitually. Does it feel unfamiliar to put on your pants and jacket this way?

- Brush your teeth, your hair and your dog with your non-dominant hand.

- Use your non-dominant hand to control your computer mouse, pet your dog, unlock a door, play tug with your dog, stir the soup, eat, and pick things up. How many things can you do with this hand? Can you write and draw with it? Pick a time when you are not rushed to explore using it.

- Wear your watch on your other wrist.

- Walk backwards.

---

[27] For wonderfully engaging and informative books on human and canine body language, refer to *The Other End of the Leash* and *For the Love of a Dog*, both by Patricia McConnell, Ph.D. For more information, visit www.PatriciaMcConnell.com.

- Learn a new skill.

- Notice if you lead with the same leg when you climb stairs. If so, alternate which leg you use on the first step.

- If you must carry your purse on your shoulder, switch to the non-habitual shoulder at least some of the time. Better yet, try carrying a light bag that crosses your torso.

- Stand on one foot as you brush your teeth and dry your hair. Or do squats. Or do one-legged squats!

- Hold your phone or tablet in your other hand.

- Take a different route to the market.

- Put on new music and dance around your living room.

- Notice how you habitually sit. Do you cross your legs? If so, does one leg feel more comfortable when it's on top? Do you tuck your legs under you? We tend to have very ingrained sitting habits, some of which can contribute to physical difficulties. Try sitting with your feet on the floor and your weight balanced.[28]

- Learn a new language. Or even a few words in a new language.

Involve more senses in everyday activities. Youngsters don't just look at things, they explore them with other senses too. *Embrace youthful playfulness, curiosity and wonder.* Where it's appropriate, focus on how things feel, sound, smell and taste. Keeping safety in mind, you might explore doing some things with your eyes closed, such as:

---

[28] The exercises that accompany this book can help you learn to sit, stand and move in a more comfortable, healthy way. For more exercises, visit www.DebonoMoves.com/Products.

- Eating. (Do you usually eat food without really tasting and savoring it? Try chewing for a longer time, putting your fork down after each mouthful. With your eyes closed, you'll really taste and smell the food. The bonus is that you'll probably be satisfied with less food.)

- Brushing your teeth. (Add using your non-dominant hand and/or standing on one foot for an even richer sensory experience.)

- Grooming and doing *Debono Moves* with your dog. (Notice how your sense of touch is enhanced when you close your eyes.)

- Unlocking your front door.

- Using your computer keyboard.

- Dressing and undressing.

Think Yourself Younger

Just as improving your movement enhances youthfulness and vitality, so too does refining the quality of your thoughts. Your inner dialogue, just like your movement, can become habitual and rigid. You can get so used to feeling worry, judgment, guilt, anxiety, or frustration that you believe your situation justifies those feelings. But could it be that those thoughts are just another *habit*?

Your body and emotions are intimately connected. You wouldn't have a feeling without a physical body to support it. To change your emotional patterns, it's best to be aware of your bodily sensations too.[29]

---

[29] Dogs' emotions are also linked to their physical bodies. This is why many people report that their dogs are more confident, social and "trainable" after having *Debono Moves* sessions. When dogs are able to relax and feel confidence in their bodies, their emotions can follow suit.

If you find yourself worried, anxious, frustrated, critical or angry, notice how your body feels. Is your breathing shallow or deep? Or are you holding your breath? What do your neck muscles feel like? What are eyes and mouth doing? Are you furrowing your brow? Frowning? It's unlikely that you are smiling!

Changing what you are doing with your body can alter your emotional state. According to author Ron Gutman, smiling can make you healthier.[30] When you smile, the levels of stress-enhancing hormones like cortisol, adrenaline, and dopamine are reduced; while mood-enhancing hormones like endorphin increase. Your blood pressure may also be lowered. You don't even have to have a reason to smile. Just the act of smiling changes the way your body *feels*.

Think about how your body feels when you are joyful. How do you breathe? How do your fingers and toes feel? Is your stomach tight or relaxed? How about your neck and back? What expression is on your face? Mold your body to a joyful state and sense how your emotion changes.

Now pay attention to your inner dialogue and notice the mental habits that no longer serve you. For example, when a new situation arises, do you immediately look for potential *problems,* rather than *opportunities?* Do you catastrophize? That habit may prevent you from enjoying all life has to offer. When you notice yourself doing this, take a deep breath and smile. Then think of all the *wonderful* things that could arise from the new situation. These steps can help you change your habit.

Feeling powerful and vital means that you are not at the mercy of thoughts and actions that sabotage you. Instead, you use your mind to *enrich* your life. If you find yourself immersed in anxious or critical thoughts, replace them with optimistic ones, even for a little while. You can tell yourself that you'll go back to worrying in ten minutes. In the

---

[30] *Smile, The Astonishing Powers of a Simple Act,* by Ron Gutman, TED books, Kindle Single

meantime, embody joy. Feel genuine appreciation for some-one or something. Look for the good in whatever situation is stressing you.

Gratitude generates a positive feeling and promotes well-being.[31] You may even start to feel happy and hopeful, and perhaps you'll come up with a solution for the problem that was bothering you.

Shifting your emotional state can change how you perceive the world, and you may find that events in your life begin to support your new, positive viewpoint.[32] Remember, if your mind is not propelling you forward in the direction you wish, change course! *Your mental flexibility is at least as important as your physical flexibility in feeling youthful.*

Tuning in to your body can help you achieve mental flexibility. By directing your attention to your physical sensations, the exercises in this book can center your mind and guide you to present-moment awareness.[33]

---

[31] There have been numerous studies showing a correlation between gratitude and wellness.

According to research published on www.HeartMath.org, generating a state of appreciation appears to improve cardiac function, regulate blood pressure and enhance immune response. "Heart-focused, sincere, positive feeling states boost the immune system, while negative emotions may suppress the immune response for up to six hours following the emotional experience." – from *The Physiological and Psychological Effects of Compassion and Anger,* 1995, Rein, Atkinson and McCraty.

[32] The suggestions in this book are not intended to replace psychiatric care. Please consult a physician if you suffer from depression or other mental illness. For healthy people, it can be beneficial to receive customized guidance in developing mental flexibility. My husband, Gary Waskowsky, helps people transform their limiting movements, thoughts and beliefs. You can learn more about Gary's work at www.GaryWaskowsky.com. See Resources at the back of the book for more information.

[33] "There is one thing that, when cultivated and regularly practiced, leads to deep spiritual intention, to peace, to mindfulness and clear comprehension, to vision and knowledge, to a happy life here and now, and to the culmination of wisdom and awakening. And what is that one thing? It is mindfulness centered on the body." – *The Buddha*

Last, but certainly not least, let this bit of information inspire you. Dogs are sensitive to our emotions, and it's not uncommon for them to mirror our internal state. This means that joy and optimism will benefit both you and your dog. And that's something we can all smile about!

Key Points of Chapter Five

- Dogs, like humans, sometimes move poorly out of habit.

- It is important to recognize the *cause* of a movement problem so that you can interrupt the vicious cycle of pain and limitation.

- Unbalanced movement, where one or more areas are chronically overused, can lead to pain, injury and/or arthritis. Balanced movement is healthy, anti-aging and can enhance athletic performance. Plus, it feels better!

- The less pressure you use, the more you and your dog will feel. The more one feels, the more one can improve.

- Small, light movements can help the brain recognize that improvement is possible and preferred.

- Pleasure and safety stimulate learning. Associate healthy, balanced movement with comfort, not force.

- Refrain from using expressions such as "good leg" and "bad leg." Describing your dog, or yourself, in those terms can leave a lasting imprint of limitation and preclude full healing.

- Positive reinforcement can help an excited, anxious or distracted dog learn to be calm and focused.

- Habits can limit you mentally and physically.

- Mental flexibility is at least as important as physical flexibility in feeling youthful.

- Non-habitual thoughts and movements promote mental and physical flexibility, enhancing youthfulness and vitality.

- Dogs often mirror our emotional state. When you feel better, your dog feels better!

Chapter Six: From Hip Dysplasia to Agility

Painful hips, stiff hips, dysplastic hips and arthritic hips. Many people worry about their dogs' hips at some point. And as dog lovers themselves age, they may notice that their *own* hips are not as flexible or comfortable as they once were.

Many will simply accept these limitations as inevitable aspects of aging, but what if you are no longer able to take your dog on a nice, long walk? Did that get your attention? And is hip trouble *really* inevitable?

If you'd like to help your dog – and yourself – have flexible, happy hips for as long as possible, please read on. I hope you find this chapter food for thought. And comfort for hips.

A Young Dog Overcomes Hip Dysplasia

Emma was even more energetic than your typical Border Collie pup. And if you've spent any time around Border Collies, you know that is saying a lot! Strikingly marked, the active black-and-white puppy enlivened Akiko and Michael's household from the minute they brought her home. Given the dog's naturally high drive, Akiko had hopes of entering Emma in canine agility competitions when she matured. But that dream appeared to be dashed when the seven-month-old puppy was diagnosed with severe hip dysplasia. The radiographs looked pretty grim, with the left hip being particularly loose. Both hips had a positive Ortolani sign, which indicates hip joint laxity and is part of the diagnostic procedure for canine hip dysplasia.

More than one veterinarian felt that the only way to give the young dog a chance at a pain-free life was by doing triple pelvic osteotomy (TPO) surgery on the left hip. But Akiko had concerns about her dog undergoing surgery. For one thing, she didn't think that her exuberant young dog could handle the long period of post-surgical confinement. Another factor was that Akiko had been down this road before. Her beloved Akita, a gentle soul named Winnie, had undergone hip dysplasia surgery as a youngster. And while the surgery repaired her hips, the changes it created in her structure seemed to adversely affect her knees and back, leaving Winnie with difficulties in her hind legs throughout her long life. Understandably, Akiko was reluctant to risk this happening to her young Border Collie, Emma.

Debono Moves is part of a team approach to managing hip dysplasia.

Keeping her dog's well-being uppermost in her mind, Akiko opted to support Emma using conservative management and alternative therapies. A diligent researcher, petite, raven-haired Akiko employed a team approach to help her Border Collie. Her veterinarian incorporated chiropractic, laser acupuncture[34], and other holistic methods. Akiko had always provided her dog with a professionally-balanced, home-prepared diet designed for a growing puppy. That diet was now modified to meet *adult* nutrient levels to slow the young Border Collie's growth. Emma's diet was also supplemented with herbs and nutraceuticals to support joint and bone health. In addition, Akiko asked me to give private *Debono Moves* sessions to Emma to help mitigate the effects of her hip dysplasia.

Would changing the way the young dog moved stimulate healthier hip joints?

Although I understood that hip dysplasia is often genetically predestined, I wanted to improve the young dog's

---

[34] Laser acupuncture uses cold lasers, rather than needles, to treat acupuncture points.

odds of staying sound and active. I began to wonder if changing how Emma moved would stimulate her body to develop healthier hip joints. After all, *form follows function.* If I could help improve her *function* (ability to walk, run, etc.), would her *form* (structure) improve as well? Could the pup's hip joints, which were still growing, develop a better fit between the "ball" and "socket"?

A tall order, for sure. But I knew that at the very least, *Debono Moves* could help the young dog move more comfortably *despite* hip dysplasia. At the most, it might stimulate the development of healthier hip joints.

One strategy I used with Emma was to *chunk down* the function of walking into small pieces. In other words, I thought about the individual movements of a dog's body that, when strung together, result in walking. By working with each piece of this walking "puzzle," Emma wouldn't feel the need to protect her hips, and would be more likely to learn healthier ways to move.

For example, when a dog walks, she has to push against the ground with her paws. That seems simple enough. But exactly *how* she does this can determine the comfort and efficiency of her gait. Does she press more with the inside of her foot? The outside? Are her toes stiff or yielding? Does one paw press harder than the others? These are the types of distinctions I look for when I watch a dog move, since the way a dog uses her paws affects her knees, hips, spine, shoulders and neck. So, with Emma lying on her side, I gently wiggled and pushed through her toes and paw pads.

The novelty of these gentle paw movements reminded the Border Collie that she didn't have to be stuck in her habitual way of using her feet. She could, instead, choose more efficient options. After all, the brain seeks efficiency. It just sometimes needs to be reminded that options exist.[35] When I

---

[35] Please refer to "When Good Habits Go Bad," in Chapter Five, to learn why dogs and humans can get stuck in unhealthy movement habits.

delicately moved her feet, I was simply suggesting new choices. Whether or not her brain adopted those new movement possibilities would be up to Emma. But this I knew: *if the dog changed the way she used her paws, she would change the way movement traveled up her legs and through her hip joints.* Her nervous system would register this change in locomotion[36].

With Emma still on her side, I brought in other components of walking, including bending and straightening her leg joints, flexing and extending her spine, and moving her ribcage, shoulder blades, neck, head and tail. Then I began to link these movements together, so that Emma's nervous system could recognize the role they played in her walking.

I wanted to give Emma the experience of moving as if she didn't have hip dysplasia.

In addition, I thought about how the Border Collie would move if she *didn't* have hip dysplasia. How would her leg joints respond to weight and movement? How differently would she move her spine? With Emma both lying down and standing up, I gently pressed through different parts of her skeleton to simulate, as best I could, how she might move without the encumbrance of hip dysplasia. I hoped that this rudimentary "blueprint" would awaken something in her nervous system and initiate improvements in her body awareness and functioning[37].

---

[36] Joint movements activate receptors that relay information to the nervous system regarding limb movement, joint angle and muscle tension. This information is used to coordinate movement.

[37] If a dog has a hip problem, it is likely that the dog has learned to compensate for the painful hip by tensing muscles around the hip joints and spine, among other places. Even in a healed injury, the body may continue to contract these muscles out of habit. By gently pressing through the pelvis, I initiate movement into the body while bypassing the legs entirely. This means that the dog has no reason to tighten the muscles that would protect against potentially painful hips, since the hips are not involved. Thus the dog has the sensory experience of movement, but free of its usual interference. Such pleasurable experiences are sometimes enough for a dog's nervous system to recognize that its habitual contractions are no longer serving a useful purpose, and can release them. This strategy can be applied to many situations, not just hip difficulties.

**It was important to relieve the strain
throughout the dog's body.**

As always, I kept *all* of Emma in mind as I worked with her. Dogs with hip dysplasia (or any hind limb soreness), commonly stress their shoulder, back and pelvic muscles to compensate for the discomfort or weakness in their hind legs. I used *Debono Moves* to help relieve the strain in those overworked areas, and helped Emma be more comfortable and balanced overall.

Just in case you are picturing me working with a relaxed, somnolent dog, let me share my reality! Emma, despite the diagnosis of hip dysplasia, continued to be very energetic. That meant that I had to be flexible in our sessions, as the vibrant young dog didn't always want to lie still. But dogs don't *have* to lie still for *Debono Moves* to be effective. When I work with very antsy dogs, their humans often call me the day after the session. With surprise in their voice, they tell me how much better their dog is moving. They confess to having thought that we hadn't accomplished much since their dog was distracted during the session. I remind them that although we could probably progress faster with a relaxed dog, even a distracted dog will typically benefit from *Debono Moves.*

The Border Collie became calmer and more relaxed as time went on, due largely to Akiko's patience in teaching Emma that lying still and being handled would earn her yummy treats. Akiko also supported her dog's progress by practicing specific *Debono Moves* that I taught her in between my sessions with Emma. Soon the young Border Collie realized how nice it felt to lie still and enjoy hands-on attention! Emma still got excitable when I visited her home, but we accomplished more and more at each session.

**X-rays reveal a surprising change in the
Border Collie's hips.**

As the months went by, the young dog became stronger and more balanced in her movement and development. Emma's hips were X-rayed again, almost a year after the diagnosis of hip dysplasia. Take a look at the radiographs to see what a difference a year makes! Pay special attention to how Emma's left hip joint (which is on the right side of each photo) fits into its hip socket. The disparity between the two X-rays is quite dramatic.

In the first one, taken in October of 2010, the left hip is obviously loose, and there are signs of arthritic changes.

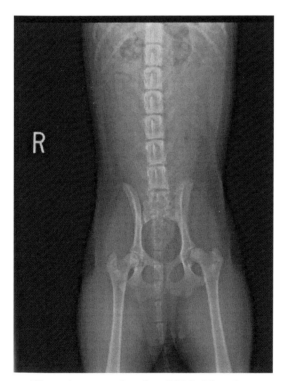

X-ray image – October 2010: Note how loosely Emma's left femur (which is on the right side as you're looking at the X-ray) fits into the socket.

The second radiograph, taken in September 2011, shows the head of each femur now fitting nicely into its hip socket, and the veterinarian said there is no longer evidence of arthritis. This was, of course, exciting and fantastic news!

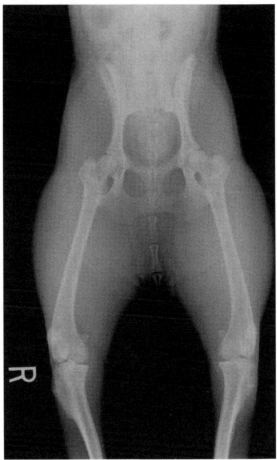

X-ray image – September 2011: Note how securely the left femur now fits into the socket!

The third photo is Emma's radiograph from September 2012. It again shows a dog with healthy hips. And as icing on the cake, the Orthopedic Foundation for Animals (OFA) gave two-year-old Emma's hips a rating of "Good." This was very surprising results for a dog whose "only option" had been surgery!

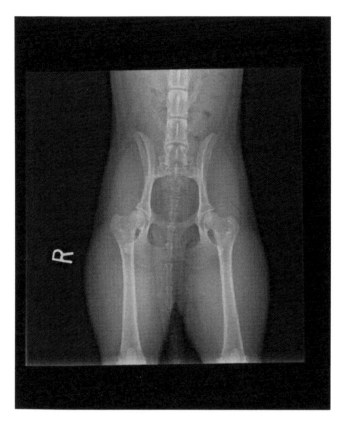

X-ray image – September 2012: Emma's hips
earned her a rating of "Good" from the OFA.

With her dog's soundness more secure, Akiko and Emma happily began canine agility training, an activity that seemed out of reach when the young dog was first diagnosed.

Since a holistic veterinarian and a canine nutritionist also contributed to Emma's care, we have no way of knowing what exact role *Debono Moves* played in the Border Collie's recovery from hip dysplasia. What we do know is that a veterinary orthopedist said that Emma's hips would never improve. And yet Emma's X-rays – and more importantly, her ability to run and play – tell a very different story. My feeling is that *all* of the modalities, including *Debono Moves,* helped support this young dog's development of healthy hip joints and contributed to her wonderful and surprising recovery.

But at the end of the day, I give the greatest credit to Akiko and her husband Michael. Their steadfast dedication to their vibrant dog is inspiring. Akiko's patient commitment to do her *Debono Moves* homework with her exuberant Border Collie helped improve her dog's body awareness and functioning, taught her how to be calm and relaxed, and deepened their strong bond.

Managing Hip Dysplasia in the Active Dog

Juliette, a black-and-white Border Collie cross, excelled at both canine agility and flyball.[38] This canine athlete competed until well into her senior years, despite being diagnosed with hip dysplasia. Some dogs with hip dysplasia get along just fine as youngsters, but develop arthritic hips and other difficulties as they age, especially if they are very active. Juliette's human, Vicki, understood this. That's why she took steps to keep her dog as healthy and pain-free as possible, while

---

[38] Flyball is a fast-paced, competitive canine sport. Flyball races match two teams of four dogs each, racing side-by-side over a 51-foot course of hurdles. Each dog must run in relay fashion down the jumps, trigger a flyball box to release a ball, retrieve the ball, and return over the jumps. The next dog is released to run the course but can't cross the start/finish line until the previous dog has returned over all four jumps and reached the start/finish line. The first team to have all four dogs finish the course without error wins the heat. View a video of this canine sport at www.coastalexpressflyball.com.

still allowing Juliette to participate in the activities she enjoyed so much.

Besides giving her dog a balanced, raw diet and regular veterinary care, Vicki enlisted me to give *Debono Moves* sessions to Juliette. Vicki wanted to minimize complications from the hip dysplasia, such as the weak hind legs, stiff spines and sore shoulders that are common in afflicted dogs. Using many of the same strategies I employed with Emma, we helped keep Juliette moving freely and comfortably for many years.

Juliette was able to run and play with Border Collie intensity for a long time, before passing away at 16½ years old. This loyal dog with the huge heart left a big impression on all she met, and she is greatly missed.

How to Help an Anxious or Distracted Dog

I never thought I would be doing something behind my own back! But there I was, sitting on the floor with my arms held behind me, delicately lifting the spinal muscles of a very shy dog. The black Lab mix, whose name was Blossom, was so anxious about strangers that she wouldn't remain still if I faced her. It was simply too much pressure for her to handle. But turning my back to her did the trick.

As Blossom felt the relief and pleasure that working with the muscles can evoke, she began to relax. Little by little, I turned my body so that I was sideways to her. Eventually I was able to face her. It helped immensely that her human reinforced her calm behavior with yummy treats, which helped the dog develop a positive outlook about being touched.[39] Over the course of several sessions, the young dog overcame her anxiety, and she began to enjoy our time together.

---

[39] Positive reinforcement training can be a wonderful way to teach shy or exuberant dogs that lying still and being handled can be a rewarding experience. To learn more, consult a qualified dog trainer who is committed to using positive reinforcement and/or visit www.whole-dog-journal.com for articles on teaching dogs how to calmly and happily accept handling.

As *Debono Moves* helped Blossom enhance her movement and confidence in her body, her emotional confidence flourished too. It was a happy day when Blossom entered my office and contentedly flopped down on the dog mat without even being asked!

The following checklist will give you some suggestions if your dog seems anxious or distracted while you are practicing *Debono Moves*:

1. Make sure that a qualified veterinarian has recently examined your dog. It is essential that you rule out the possibility that a medical problem is causing your dog discomfort.

2. Is this a time of day when your dog would normally be getting fed or going for a walk? If so, it may be wise to reschedule *Debono Moves* practice for a time when your dog is more likely to be relaxed and not anticipating food, play or a walk. Refer to Chapter Three, "Make it All About You and Your Dog," to be sure you are creating the best environment for your dog's *Debono Moves* experience.

3. Your dog may be telling you that it's time for a break. When you are first learning *Debono Moves,* do it only for a few minutes at a time. As you gain confidence and skill, your dog will let you know that she wants longer sessions. In the meantime, offer your dog some water and give her a chance to stretch her legs.

4. Allow your dog to pick the position he is most relaxed in. If he is showing signs of stress while lying on his side, perhaps that side is not comfortable at the moment. See if changing sides helps. Or encourage him to lie down like a sphinx, sit up, or even stand. Let it be his choice. While you can gently ask and encourage him to be in a certain position, please do not force your dog. Honor your dog's

comfort. Oftentimes I have found that the dog will then relax and voluntarily turn onto his side quite contentedly![40]

5. Is your dog continually rolling onto his side for you to rub his belly? It takes some dogs a while before they realize that this isn't about tummy rubs! It's generally best to separate *Debono Moves* practice from your normal petting and scratching. Be patient and consistent. Be assured that dogs do eventually figure it out. They also will come to realize that *Debono Moves* are as pleasurable as a belly rub. And you will feel good knowing that you are helping improve your dog's freedom of movement and well-being while giving them a pleasurable experience.

6. Lighten up! *Debono Moves* should be done very gently. If your dog objects to your touch, try reducing your pressure. A lot.

7. Be mindful of your body position. For many dogs, leaning over them is stressful. So is staring directly at them. If your dog is uncomfortable, change your position. Try sitting sideways to your dog, for example. Or scoot back a little to give your dog more space. As my story about Blossom illustrated, dogs are sensitive to the pressure we inadvertently exert on them. This is especially true of dogs who are new to your family.

8. Do *Connected Breathing* with your dog until he fully relaxes again.[41] This will help ensure that you are calm and breathing in a relaxed way too. Remember that our dogs often mirror our own internal state. Make sure you are not so intent on "getting it right" that you inadvertently project stress onto your dog. *Debono Moves* is designed to be pleasurable for dog and human, so have fun!

9. Talk soothingly to your dog. The voice can be a useful aid in calming a fearful dog, but avoid high-pitched "baby

---

[40] See Cassie's story in Chapter Three.

[41] See *Connected Breathing* in Chapter Two.

talk." Some dogs prefer silence during *Debono Moves,* so try being quiet. Notice how your dog reacts to your voice or silence, and act accordingly.

10. Put your hands on a different part of your dog's body. Perhaps your dog has discomfort or anticipates discomfort in the area you were touching.

11. I have found it helpful to let my hands hover over areas that a dog anticipates pain in. This is referred to as working off body. By keeping your hands a few inches away from the body, the dog gains confidence that you are not going to hurt her. I may start as much as several inches away, then gradually bring my hand closer and closer as long as the dog is not showing any sign of stress. I like to come in so gradually that the transition from hovering to touching the body is virtually unnoticed by the dog.

When I am working off body, I don't simply hover my hands over the dog. Instead, I imagine that I am contacting the dog's body and doing a specific *Debono Move.* I imagine it feeling easy and comfortable for the dog. I make the experience seem as real as possible by imagining the feel of the dog's hair, muscles, etc. I have found that this soft, focused attention helps dogs accept my contact **and** to move more freely when I do touch them. I often use it with dogs who are anxious, infirm and/or recovering from injury.[42]

Taking the time to ensure your dog's comfort is essential to building your dog's confidence and trust in your relationship. Some dogs, especially those that have been abused or painfully poked and prodded for medical reasons, need to time to recognize how good *Debono Moves* can feel!

---

[42] Another related strategy has provided interesting feedback. I sometimes imagine that I'm leaving my hands on an area when I move to another part of the body. I can't tell you what dogs feel when I do this, but several humans have commented to me that they felt as if I had four hands! Their comments were unsolicited and they had no knowledge that I was using my imagination in this way.

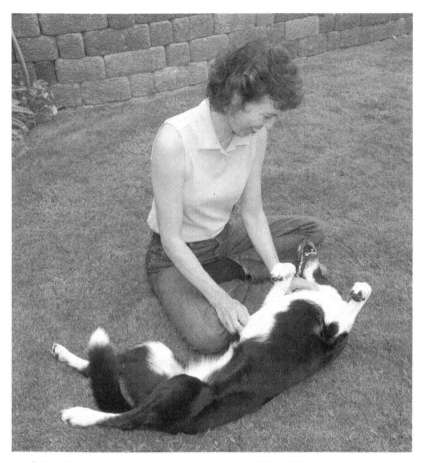

Maggie wants me to scratch her belly! This high-energy dog is new to *Debono Moves* and wasn't quite sure what to do. I stayed patient and relaxed myself, which helped calm her. She was eventually able to notice how pleasurable *Debono Moves* felt and she relaxed into it. Stay patient and don't try to force your dog to lie still.

Human Exercise #8: Making Time for Freer Hips

Benefits: Many people complain of sore or tight hips. By refining the movement of your pelvis, this exercise can help release restrictions around your hip joints and lower back, leading to happier hips.

Listen to the audio recording of this exercise by going to www.debonomoves.com/dog-book and typing in the password *free*.

The exercise is printed and illustrated in Chapter Eight.

Human Exercise #9: Sitting on a Clock

Benefits: This exercise can help release restrictions around your hip joints and lower back, leading to happier hips and more comfortable sitting and walking.

This exercise can also improve your ability to do the *Debono Moves* that require you to move your pelvis lightly in a circle as you work with your dog.

Listen to the audio recording of this exercise by going to www.debonomoves.com/dog-book and typing in the password *free*.

The exercise is printed and illustrated in Chapter Eight.

Muscle Lifts

View a video of Mary teaching *Muscle Lifts* and *Muscle Rolls* by going to www.debonomoves.com/dog-book and typing in the password *free*.

Benefits may include:

- Improves body awareness.
- Reduces muscle tension and stiffness.
- Relaxes and comforts your dog.
- Allows you to feel where your dog may be habitually contracting muscles.
- Helps you coordinate your movement more efficiently, reducing wear and tear on your body.

Muscle Lifts provide hands-on support to relieve sore, tight muscles and promote a calm, relaxed state.

Position: *Muscle Lifts* can be done in any position, but are most often done with the dog lying down.

Muscle Lifts can be done almost anywhere on your dog's body, and the technique itself is quite simple. You use your hands to gently support (lift) your dog's muscles. Depending on the size of the area you are working with, you can use either your whole hand(s), a portion of your hand(s), or just your fingertips. There is no one "correct" way to do it. *I encourage you to experiment and notice what feels most soothing and pleasant for your dog.*

Practicing *Muscle Lifts* on yourself can help you fine-tune your technique. With your right arm lying comfortably across your abdomen, put your left hand on the muscle just below your right elbow. Have your whole left hand in soft contact with your right forearm.

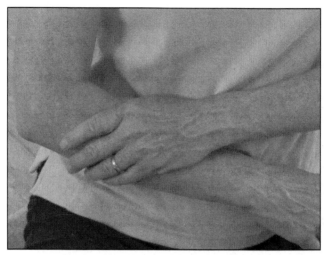

Gently push up the muscle so that it moves
toward your elbow.

Keeping your whole left hand (palm and fingers) in contact with your right forearm, gently push up the muscle of your right forearm so that it moves a little bit toward your right elbow. Hold that position for several seconds. Make it a soft, supportive pressure. You should feel your right forearm muscle move a little bit. Take a few breaths, then very slowly release your pressure. Move to a slightly different spot on your arm and repeat the lift.

Notice how much tension is in your left hand as you do the *Muscle Lift*. Become aware of how you create the movement. Is your hand doing all the work or is there movement in your left shoulder? Try it both ways. First, have all the movement come from your left hand while your left shoulder stays passive. Then move your left shoulder forward a little bit so that it pushes your left hand. Can you feel how this allows your left hand to stay soft and sensitive? Can you feel more when your hand is relaxed?

Experiment with how to make the *Muscle Lift* feel pleasant. Try it on your upper arm, your thigh, your calf, etc.

129

Explore how using different parts of your hand changes the sensation. Did you try using just your fingertips?

Make sure you practice with both your dominant and non-dominant hands. Which one is more sensitive?

Practice with a human friend too and invite feedback. The idea is to have the *Muscle Lift* be an exercise in awareness for both the giver and receiver.

Practice with your dog. This exercise explains how to do *Muscle Lifts* on your dog's legs. With your dog lying comfortably on his side, sit facing his outstretched legs.

Shoulder Blade

Let's assume that your dog is lying on his right side, with his head facing to your left. Gently support the bottom of your dog's left shoulder with your left hand. Place your right hand on your dog's shoulder blade. Use your right hand to lightly push up the soft tissue on your dog's shoulder blade. Use only gentle pressure. Notice if you are pressing mostly with the heel of your hand or some other part. *Distribute the pressure evenly throughout your hand so that your dog can feel the support you are providing, rather than noticing a sensation of pressure.* Hold this lift for several seconds and then release it slowly. You can repeat the lift a few times on the same area if your dog is comfortable.

Move your hand an inch or so away and repeat the lift. When you and your dog are first doing *Muscle Lifts,* you might only do a few. But as your skill improves and your dog begins to feel the muscular relief you are providing, he will probably be quite content to have you do *Muscle Lifts* all over his body, for as long as you'd like!

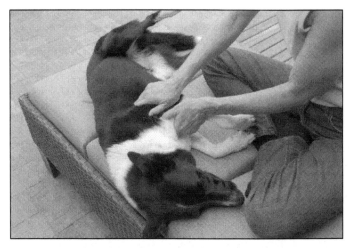

I mold my hands around Maggie's shoulder,
providing a supportive lift to the muscles.

Lower Leg

You can use two hands to softly envelop your dog's leg
and lift up the soft tissue. Hold this lift for several seconds
and release very gradually.

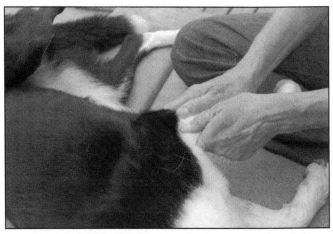

My two hands lift the muscles between Maggie's
wrist and elbow.

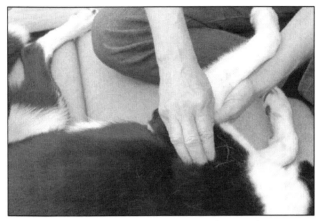

The fingertips of my right hand lift muscles on
the upper foreleg. My left hand supports her leg
by comfortably holding her elbow.

Hindquarters

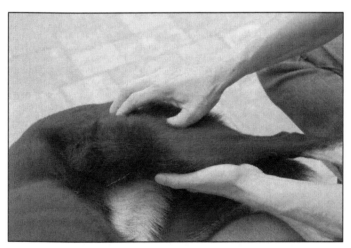

I use the fingertips of my right hand to delicately lift
muscles on Maggie's hindquarters, while my left
hand supports her leg.

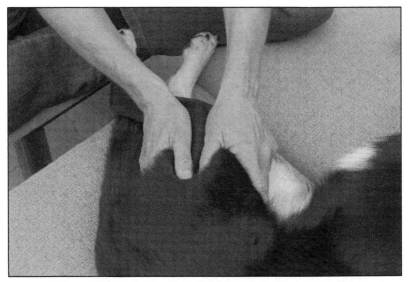

I'm using both hands to lift Maggie's thigh muscles.

Muscle Rolls

View a video of Mary teaching *Muscle Lifts* and *Muscle Rolls* by going to www.debonomoves.com/dog-book and typing in the password *free*.

Benefits may include:

- Improves canine body awareness.

- Reduces muscle tension and stiffness.

- Relaxes and comforts your dog.

- Allows you to feel where your dog may be habitually contracting muscles.

- Improves your ability to use your back and hips, making your movement comfortable and reducing wear and tear.

The ***Muscle Roll*** is a useful variation on the *Muscle Lift*. Please practice the *Muscle Lift* if you haven't done that already. It's also important that you do the Human Exercise #8, *Making Time for Freer Hips,* and Human Exercise #9, *Sitting on a Clock,* in Chapter Eight before you do this move with your dog.

Position: The *Muscle Roll* can be done in any position, but is commonly done with the dog lying down.

Like the *Muscle Lift,* the *Muscle Roll* can be done almost anywhere on your dog's body. You use your hands to gently support (lift) your dog's muscles and then **you lightly roll the soft tissue in a circle**. Depending on the size of the area you are working with, you can use either your whole hand(s), a portion of your hand(s), or just your fingertips. Just like a *Muscle Lift,* there is no one "correct" way to do it. *I encourage you to experiment and notice what feels most soothing and pleasant for your dog.*

Practice with yourself first. Put the palm of your left hand on the meaty part of your right forearm, below your elbow. Let your entire left hand mold itself to this area, then gently press the muscle towards your elbow, so that you are doing a *Muscle Lift. Maintaining a light pressure, move the muscle around in a circle.* Make a few clockwise circles and then a few counterclockwise circles. This is a *Muscle Roll.*

Notice how you create this movement. Is your hand doing all the work or is there movement in your left shoulder? Let's try it both ways. First, have all the movement come from your left hand while your left shoulder stays passive. Next, initiate the movement from your left shoulder by making light, easy, smooth circles with your left shoulder. How does this feel? Most people prefer this sensation. They also report that the smoother their left shoulder circles become, the nicer the *Muscle Roll* feels.

Switch which arm you are using and try it again. How is it different when you use this arm? Does one seem easier? Can you do the movement so that both sides are equally easy and light?

In addition to this being a good exercise to improve your own movement and body awareness, it also illustrates how the more easily and efficiently you learn to move, the more you can help your dog!

Now that you have the idea, find a human friend and practice with each other. The feedback you receive can help you refine your touch.

Practice with your dog. Sit comfortably and lightly hold your hands in front of you with your elbows bent. Slowly move your pelvis around in a circle, like you learned in Exercise #5, "Stirring the Soup," and Exercise #9, "Sitting on a Clock." Can you feel your arms moving a little bit? It's most likely a small, subtle movement. Do several circles in each direction until you are satisfied that you can feel your arms respond to the movement of your pelvis. Now ask your dog to lie down on her side.

Refer to the section earlier in this chapter and review the explanation of how to do *Muscle Lifts* with your dog. Next, do a *Muscle Lift* on your dog's shoulder. Maintaining the lift, roll your dog's muscle around in a circle, just like you did on your forearm. That's a *Muscle Roll*.

Notice how you do this. Are you moving only your hands? Is your pressure light or are you squeezing your dog? Is there movement in your shoulders? Do you feel your pelvis moving? *Deliberately move your pelvis in a slow, easy circle and feel what happens.* Does this help your dog's muscle roll lightly and easily?

Move to various parts of your dog's front and hind legs and do *Muscle Rolls* at each place. Can you make the rolling happen by moving your pelvis in a circle? Does this keep your arms and hands light and soft? Explore rolling the muscles of your dog's shoulders, thighs and lower legs.

Mary's Tip:

Your arms, hands and neck, with their relatively-small, fine muscles, are designed to *sense and direct movement.* The body parts with large muscles, such as the trunk and buttocks, are equipped to do most of the work of *moving* your body. But many people habitually overuse the small-muscled parts of the body. This can lead to pain, stiffness, wear and tear injuries and fatigue.

As you go about your day, think about where you can release unnecessary effort or feelings of tension. Be curious, rather than judgmental. For example, ask yourself: *Is my jaw relaxed? Am I breathing in a full, easy way? Can I relax my eyes? Is my head free to turn easily? Can I move from my pelvis and keep my hands soft? Where else can I reduce my effort?*

The exercises in this book can help you coordinate your movement so that your large muscles do their share of the work, leading to greater efficiency and reduced wear and tear. Enhanced comfort, flexibility and stamina can be your reward.[43]

---

[43] See Resources, right after Chapter Eight, or www.DebonoMoves.com/Products for additional educational products that can help you progress even more.

Key Points of Chapter Six

- *Debono Moves* can be part of a team approach to managing hip problems.

- Since *form follows function*, improving movement may improve structure.

- "Chunk down" a problem into manageable, changeable pieces.

- *Debono Moves* can relieve the widespread tension and soreness that often accompanies orthopedic problems.

- Explore your options before accepting a limiting prognosis.

- *Debono Moves* can enhance canine athletic performance *and* behavior.

- Letting your pelvis move your arms generally feels more pleasurable to your dog than if you initiated the movement with your arms. It's also healthier for you, as it reduces wear and tear on your shoulders, elbows and hands.

- *Debono Moves* is designed so that you and your canine companion can improve your movement and well-being together.

- Be patient and creative with anxious or distracted dogs. The rewards are well worth it!

Chapter Seven: Enhancing the Life of the Older Dog

When our dogs are young, it's easy to take their health for granted. They run and play with ease and are always game for a hike up a hill or a romp on the beach. But things often change when our dogs get older. They may lose their vitality, become sore after a long game of fetch, and even become grumpy at times. That also describes a lot of humans!

Read this chapter to learn how *Debono Moves* helped two geriatric canines regain more youthful movement. These two older dogs, both suffering from painful, limited movement, regained the ability to walk unimpeded. After their sessions, the dogs were able to go on walks and enjoy family play time with their people again. I also teach exercises to help *you* move a little easier, a little younger too. I hope this chapter encourages you to take charge of your aging – and that of your dog. It's never too late to feel younger!

Geriatric Dog Learns How to Wag Her Tail Again

We all watched intently as Nancy led her geriatric Irish Setter into the room. The dog, whose name was Seana, moved with a slow, stiff gait. She held her body rigidly, was limping on her left front leg, and her tail drooped lifelessly. Nancy told the assembled group that Seana had the usual complications of getting old: arthritis and decreased vitality. She also told us that it had been over a year since she had seen her dog wag her tail.

Even a *Debono Moves* novice can make a big difference to a dog.

I assigned my student Karen to work with Seana. Although I stepped back to let them get acquainted, I remained watching from a distance to make sure that all went well. Karen, along with several other people, were participating in a week-long *Debono Moves* class, and I had asked local dog lovers to bring their canine companions for my students to work with. We had a room full of dogs, their guardians and my workshop participants.

The students had been learning about *Debono Moves* for a week. Monday through Friday they learned how to apply it to horses; Saturday they learned how those same concepts were applied to dogs; and today, Sunday, they were getting supervised, hands-on experience with dogs.

Tiny, gentle movements along a dog's spine can reawaken movement.

With Seana settled comfortably on her side on a soft mat, Karen used her fingers to delicately lift the Irish Setter's spinal muscles a tiny amount. It was an amount so small that an observer would think that Karen wasn't doing anything. Slowly and patiently, Karen's fingers traveled from the base of the red dog's skull down to the end of her feathery tail. She intended for these supportive, novel movements to relax and "wake up" all the parts of the dog's back so that Seana could use her spine more easily. Partway through the session, Karen helped the Setter turn over so she could work with her other side.

The quality of our attention facilitates the dog's improvement.

Karen also gently explored movements of Seana's ribcage, shoulders and hips. Karen used basic, but effective, *Debono Moves.* So effective, in fact, that the class cheered when the Irish Setter got up after her session and wagged her lovely plume of a tail. This dog, who had entered the room in a stiff, halting fashion, now moved with a spring in her step. Even her limp was gone!

Her human, Nancy, could hardly believe the difference in her dog. The degeneration and lack of vitality, which many believed to be irreversible, was considerably reduced. It is worth repeating that the woman who gave the session to Seana had only been introduced to *Debono Moves* a week earlier. After teaching *Debono Moves* for over 20 years, I am still joyful when I see how easily people can learn how to help animals.[44]

Karen did only a few *Debono Moves* with the Irish Setter, but she did them slowly, patiently and with the utmost attention to the dog. Her session with Seana was a beautiful example of how giving our full attention to doing a few basic *Debono Moves* can improve the quality of life of our canine partners.

Hope for an Older Dog Who Could No Longer Stand

Ron and Paula had a painful decision to make. Their beloved Malamute, Nikki, had been gradually losing the ability to walk or even stand. Her hindquarters were weak, and her left front leg had begun to knuckle over when she put weight on it. Her tail, which had once been held aloft, now hung down limply. Nikki could not stand up long enough to eat on her own, so Ron and Paula fed their beloved dog by hand while she was lying down.

Ron and Paula had always enjoyed the long walks they took with their 11½-year-old Malamute. Now it saddened them to think that Nikki's days of roaming the neighborhood were over.

---

[44] *Debono Moves* was formerly known as the *SENSE Method*.

The Malamute's veterinarian took X-rays and did blood work, trying to get at the source of the dog's problem. The radiographs showed that Nikki had arthritis in her spine, but that didn't fully explain her decline. Both steroids and non-steroidal anti-inflammatories (NSAIDs) were tried, but the medications didn't help Nikki's condition. Ron and Paula feared their options had run out.

They were desperate for one last chance to save their Malamute.

The couple still held onto a shred of hope that they could find a solution to their dog's problem, so they continued their research. It was during one of these online searches that Ron discovered my website. After reading about other dogs that I helped, Ron contacted me immediately.

I heard the emotion in Ron's voice as he spoke about Nikki's decline. It seemed that he and Paula had made the decision that euthanasia would be in their dog's best interests if the Malamute didn't improve soon. I could tell how much Nikki was loved, and it broke my heart to imagine what Ron and his wife were facing. I explained to Ron that I did not know if I could make a big enough difference for his dog. I simply couldn't tell that in advance. Ron assured me that he understood that I could not offer any guarantees, but he wanted to give *Debono Moves* a chance at helping Nikki before an irreversible decision was made. That left little doubt that I would have to see this Malamute very soon. Time was running out.

Even though they lived almost two hours away, Ron and Paula gently lifted the large dog into their sedan and headed to Cardiff-by-the-Sea, California. The traffic wasn't as bad as they had feared, and they arrived at our meeting place before I did. As I pulled my Honda up to the curb, my heart caught in my throat when I saw Nikki. She was lying crumpled on the lawn, with Ron and Paula kneeling by her side. Paula, petite and dark-haired, was squirting water into Nikki's mouth from a sports bottle. The Malamute could no longer drink on her own, and she depended on her people for this most basic need.

I said a silent prayer that I could help this dog. Then I got out of my car and greeted the trio. Ron, a tall and trim gentleman, helped Nikki move into my canine studio, and the large grey-and-white dog immediately rested her tired body on a comfortable mat.

Connection and support set the stage for improvement.

With Nikki lying on her side, I placed my hands lightly on her ribcage and did *Connected Breathing.*[45] After Nikki's breathing deepened and slowed, I seamlessly segued into very small *Ribcage Slides and Circles.*[46] I monitored the Malamute's breathing and expressions throughout our session, making sure that she stayed comfortable and relaxed.

As I gently touched and moved the large dog, I could feel that Nikki's muscles were tight and overworked. Her front legs had been compensating for her weakening hindquarters for several months. And her right front leg had an even larger burden ever since the Malamute's left front leg had begun to knuckle over.

Rhythmic movements can renew a stiff or ailing dog.

On all four of Nikki's limbs, I created lines of *Rhythm Circles* that went from her paws to the top of each leg.[47] The rhythmic nature of these circular movements might "reset" the

---

[45] To learn how to do *Connected Breathing*, please refer to Chapter Two.

[46] For more information on *Ribcage Slides and Circles,* please see Nicky's story in the section "A Neck Injury Doesn't Stop this Canine Athlete" in Chapter Four.

[47] For more on *Rhythm Circles,* please see Nicky's story in the section "A Neck Injury Doesn't Stop this Canine Athlete" in Chapter Four.

ailing dog's internal rhythm, while their upward supportive lift could relieve Nikki's sore, overworked muscles. I could see Nikki's grey-and-white chest rise and fall with deepened breathing. I also drew *Rhythm Circles* around each leg joint, emphasizing the support of soft tissue toward the joints. I have found that delicately working around the joints in this way is very calming to the nervous system. It also seems to help improve the articulation of the joints, probably by releasing tension in the surrounding tissue and by its overall relaxing effect.

Overusing parts of the body can lead to arthritis and other degenerative changes.

Like a great many dogs and humans, the Malamute seemed to overuse some parts of her back and underuse other parts. Over time, this habit can lead to arthritis of the spine, with which Nikki was diagnosed. To help mitigate the effects of the spinal arthritis, I wanted to stimulate her brain to use her back more fully.

Support can reduce strain and invite healing.

To do this, I used my fingers to gently lift the soft tissue adjacent to the dog's spine, working from her head to her tail, and back up to her head again. As I gently supported each small area, I imagined a healing vibration that would spread out and resonate through Nikki's entire body. The gentle, non-habitual lifts were also "waking up" parts of her spine that her brain may have tuned out, thus reducing strain on other parts. With Nikki's diagnosis of spinal arthritis, this was vital.

I recreated movements that Nikki had done when she was able to walk and run.

To help the dog integrate her new body awareness, I used my hands to do very small rounding and arching movements of her back. I was careful to make miniscule, easy movements. If I caused discomfort or anxiety, the dog would resist the movements. But if I kept the movements small and comfortable, there was a chance that Nikki would recreate them on her own.

In efficient movement, the ribcage usually moves slightly downward toward the pelvis when the back rounds, and upward toward the head when the back arches. I used my hands to gently encourage the ribcage to follow along as Nikki's spine rounded and arched. Recruiting more parts of the body could help Nikki move her back more freely.

The brain doesn't need big movements, it just needs new ideas.

Next, I thought about how the movements of the back and hindquarters were coordinated when a dog walked or ran. To simulate this coordination, I moved Nikki's pelvis and hind legs a tiny amount, tucking her hind legs underneath her when her back rounded, and a wee bit behind her when her spine arched. These movements were so small they were almost thoughts rather than actual movements. It's much more effective to use miniscule, comfortable movements rather than larger, uncomfortable ones. The brain doesn't need big movements to stimulate new neural pathways. *It just needs new ideas.* I hoped that the new kinesthetic "blueprint" my hands were providing would awaken something in Nikki's brain, reminding her of the coordination required to walk on her own.

We improved the Malamute's ability to stand and walk when she was lying down.

To add another physical clue that could help Nikki stand and walk easier, I used a CD case (any small, flat object would work) to create an *"Artificial Floor."* With Nikki still lying on her side, I held this *Artificial Floor* against the bottom of one paw. Using the CD case, I gently moved each toe, one at a time. I repeated this with all four paws. When the nervous system detects something firm and flat under the foot, the brain recognizes that as standing. This means that the *Artificial Floor* gave Nikki the *sensory experience* of standing, and could stimulate her brain to evoke the physical functions that would allow the Malamute to actually stand.[48]

Before I brought our session to a close, I put one hand on the Malamute's hip and the other on her shoulder. Then I moved both my hands in slow circles. These passive movements helped remind Nikki how the shoulder and hip on each side could move easily. Once again, novel movements like *Hip and Shoulder Circles*[49] can stimulate the brain to discover healthier movement options.

It's helpful to integrate the new movement sensations throughout the body.

To help Nikki have a better awareness of her entire body, I put one hand on the dog's pelvis and the other hand on her head, and I imagined movement travelling smoothly through her spine. Then I helped Nikki to her feet and again put my hands on her pelvis and head. As I removed my hands, I noticed that there was an improvement in the dog's balance and walking. I still didn't know how much functioning the Malamute would recover, but we were off to an optimistic start. Ron and Paula then helped Nikki back into their car for the long drive home.

Nikki is indeed the Miracle Dog!

---

[48] To learn how I used the *Artificial Floor* with other dogs, please refer to Rocky's story in Chapter Two and Sonny's story in Chapter Five. The *Artificial Floor* is often used with humans in the *Feldenkrais Method* of Somatic Education.

[49] To learn how you and your dog can benefit from *Hip and Shoulder Circles*, please refer to Chapter Five and Chapter Eight.

The next day I received an email from Ron. He wrote that Nikki had sat up in the car on the way home, looking out the window for almost 30 minutes. She had not sat up in the car in quite awhile, so that was a happy surprise. But there was even more exciting news. When Nikki got home, she ate her dinner standing up! No more eating or drinking while lying down. The Malamute was even walking around their large back yard, her tail held high! Ron, Paula and I were thrilled at Nikki's dramatic turnaround.

The Malamute quickly grew stronger and began going on short walks again. At first, Nikki wore a brace that supported her hips, but soon she didn't need it. In fact, someone who knew Nikki before her *Debono Moves* session didn't recognize the dog when she saw her walking with Ron. The woman thought that Paula and Ron had adopted a new Malamute!

Nikki, aka *"The Miracle Dog,"* now wears a happy expression as she walks and trots at a lively pace.[50] And I smile every time I think of her. This remarkable grey-and-white dog is a wonderful example of our ability to improve functioning. No matter the age, no matter the condition, some improvement is usually possible.

We can all become partners in healing with our dogs.

Even though I had no way of knowing how much progress Nikki would make that day, I knew that I could, at the very least, offer the dog *something* useful. And that is what I offer you, dear readers. We all have the ability to give our dogs, no matter how old or infirm they may be, an improved degree of comfort. We may or may not experience a dramatic turnaround like Nikki did. I realize that time marches on and

---

[50] To watch a video of Nikki, visit www.youtube.com/watch?v=HoCsl-jDqIU.

our physical bodies don't stay the same. But we can all do *something* helpful for our dogs, and for ourselves.

We must remember that we hold in our hands the ability to improve our dogs' quality of life. And ours. When we open ourselves up to the beauty and optimism of love, a love that transcends the physical body, we become partners in healing with our canine companions.

Lumbar Lifts

View a video of Mary teaching *Lumbar Lifts and Lumbar Circles* by going to www.debonomoves.com/dog-book and typing in the password *free*.

Benefits may include:

- Relieves low back stress and strain, which often accompanies hind leg problems.
- As with all *Debono Moves*, it enhances body awareness and is comforting and pleasurable for most dogs.

I was doing *Lumbar Lifts* with Rocky when we connected in such a profound way, and I have found that most dogs find it quite pleasurable.[51] I have seen it relieve lower back stress and promote freer movement. I often pair *Lumbar Lifts* with more advanced techniques.[52]

Position: You can do *Lumbar Lifts* with your dog in any position, but it is easiest to learn the technique when your dog

---

[51] *Lumbar Lifts* are also referred to as "Rocky's Relief." Read Rocky's story in Chapter Two.

[52] To learn more advanced *Debono Moves*, please see Resources immediately following Chapter Eight or visit DebonoMoves.com.

is lying flat on his side. That is the position we'll explore in this book.

Practice with your dog. Let's assume that your dog is lying on his right side. Sit behind your dog so that you are facing his tail. If you need to, modify the position so that you are comfortable. Put your right hand on your dog's lower back, to the left of his spine. *Your right hand should be just behind the back of your dog's ribcage.* You'll find that this area is more "meaty" than your dog's ribcage. Gently but securely support your dog's left hind leg with your left hand. Refer to the photo for the proper hand placement.

Using a *very gentle* pressure of your right hand, lightly press the muscle toward your dog's head. Allow your hand to mold to the contours of your dog's body, distributing the pressure evenly throughout your hand.

Hold the lift for several seconds. Don't forget to breathe! Keep your hands soft as you support your dog. Release the lift very slowly and repeat the process a few times. If your dog is comfortable, there is no need to put the hind leg down between *Lumbar Lifts*. Do a few *Lumbar Lifts* and then move on to *Lumbar Circles*, which is described on the next page.

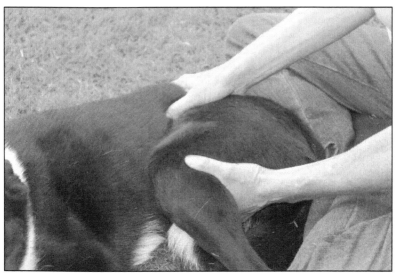

My right hand gently lifts Maggie's back muscle while my left hand supports her hind leg.

Lumbar Circles

View a video of Mary teaching *Lumbar Lifts* and *Lumbar Circles* by going to www.debonomoves.com/dog-book and typing in the password *free.*

Benefits may include:

- Enhanced flexibility and coordination.
- Can restore body confidence after an injury has healed.
- Improved flexibility and coordination of *your* back and hips too.

Here's a fun way to improve your dog's comfort, flexibility and coordination while you reap the same benefits too! Please do the human exercise #9, *Sitting on a Clock* in

Chapter Six, as well as *Lumbar Lifts* with your dog, before you do this move.

Sit comfortably and lightly hold your hands in front of you with your elbows bent. Do a few slow *pelvic circles*. Can you feel your arms moving a little bit? Do several circles in each direction until you are satisfied that you can feel your arms respond to the movement of your pelvis. Now ask your dog to lie down on her side.

Position: You can do *Lumbar Circles* with your dog in any position, but it is easiest to learn the technique when your dog is lying flat on her side. That is the position we'll explore in this book.

Practice with your dog. We'll assume that your dog is lying on her right side. As with *Lumbar Lifts* above, sit behind your dog's tail. Put your right hand on your dog's lower back, to the left of her spine. *Your hand should be just behind the back of your dog's ribcage.* Gently support your dog's left hind leg with your left hand.

Using a very gentle pressure of your right hand, do a *Lumbar Lift.* Allow your hand to mold to the contours of your dog's body, distributing the pressure evenly throughout your hand. Maintaining this support with your hand, do a few slow *Pelvic Circles.*

Your hands will lightly support your dog's muscles and your arms should be passive. As you move your pelvis in a circle, you will notice that your arms are being moved too.

Letting your pelvis move your arms generally feels more pleasurable to your dog than if you initiated the movement with your arms. It's also healthier for you, as it reduces wear and tear on shoulders, elbows and hands. As with all Debono Moves, both you and your dog can benefit when these exercises are done mindfully.

Do a few slow circles in each direction. Gradually stop your movement, pause, and remove your hands slowly. Ask

151

your dog to turn onto her other side and repeat. Notice if you sense any differences between one side and the other.

Add More Time to Your Life ... And More Life to Your Time

Have you noticed that the older we get, the faster time seems to fly by? Well, that's not your imagination. The fact is, our brains tend to process time differently as we age. The good news is that we can slow time down, or at least our perception of time.

According to neuroscientist David Eagleman, engaging in novel activities changes how the brain processes time, making it seem longer.[53] The older you get, the more familiar your experiences routinely are, and the faster your brain processes them. This rapid processing makes time appear to go swiftly.

Eagleman has found that when you engage in something unfamiliar, your brain takes a relatively long time to process the new information. The longer it takes for your brain to process something, the more extended that time period feels. Thus, non-habitual activities prevent time from slipping by. Although clock time may be the same for both routine and novel activities, your *perception* of time will be different. Non-habitual activities help you perceive time slowly, like you did when you were young, when many of your experiences were new.[54]

Debono Moves, which is chock-full of novel movements, sensations and focused attention, can help you perceive time

----

[53] David Eagleman is the author of several books, including *Incognito: The Secret Lives of the Brain.* He is a neuroscientist at Baylor's College of Medicine, Houston, Texas.

[54] For more suggestions on incorporating novelty into your life, refer to Chapter Five, "Taking Off Your Pants Can Keep You Nimble."

more fully. In addition, it provides numerous anti-aging benefits for you and your dog.

To help you get the most benefit from *Debono Moves*, I've included guidelines below. You can also apply these recommendations to dog training and many other endeavors. In short, they can help you get more out of *life*. I call them the **Seven Suggestions**.

The Seven Suggestions

1. **Feel gratitude**. Sense the love and appreciation you have for your dog. Gratitude replaces worry about the future and regret about the past, grounding you in the *now*. Such present moment awareness gives you the feeling that you have an abundance of time. Dogs love when we live in this state. Whatever time you can set aside to be with your dog, let it feel abundant. Be grateful for every precious moment.

2. **Be self-aware.** How you move, breathe and think influences your dog. Being mindful of your comfort while doing *Debono Moves* enriches the experience for you and your dog. It also helps you release the habit of stressing and straining.

3. **Cultivate pleasure.** Pleasure promotes learning while anxiety and discomfort stifle it. Keep experiences enjoyable for you and your dog. Take the time to sense pleasant moments, for they are life's riches. Find out what your dog enjoys and do more of it. Do the same for yourself too. Your mind and body – and your dog – will be the better for it.

4. **Ask questions.** When doing *Debono Moves* with your dog, you are *asking questions with your hands*. Using a

listening touch, discover what movements are easy for your dog and build on that. Do not use force. *Ask, support and suggest* rather than correct and control. When doing the human exercises, ask yourself how your movement can become lighter and easier. *Asking questions stimulates your brain to seek solutions.*

5. **Use slow, light movements.** Gentle movements heighten your sensations, making it easier for you and your dog to discover freer, healthier movement. If you notice resistance, instead of pushing through it, slow down and lighten up.

6. **Use novelty and variation.** *Debono Moves* are non-habitual and varied, thus stimulating the creation of new neural pathways. This leads to improved body awareness and easier movement. To keep you and your dog flexible in body and mind, introduce novelty and variation into your everyday life.

7. **Be open to new possibilities.**

    *   *An open mind and helpful hands can do much to change a dog's future.* Let your hands and heart transmit the sense of new possibilities to your dog, then accept that healing takes many forms and follows its own timeline.

    *   You can create new possibilities for yourself too. Instead of believing that life follows an inevitable and uncomfortable downhill slide, take action by learning healthier ways to move and think. It will influence not only how you feel today, but also 20 or more years down the road.[55] Empowered with curiosity and optimism, you can unlock your true potential!

---

[55] In addition to doing the exercises that I offer on my website and in workshops, it can be beneficial to have private sessions with a *Feldenkrais.*

Exercise #10: Better Posture Effortlessly

Benefits: Striving to obtain better posture often leads to strain, fatigue and unhealthy movement. This exercise can help you learn how to be upright without effort, eliminating the rounded back that so often develops from constant sitting and stress.

This exercise also improves the power and use of your back, leading to more coordinated, balanced movement. Discover how you can look, move and feel younger!

Listen to the audio recording of this exercise by going to www.debonomoves.com/dog-book and typing in the password *free*.

The exercise is printed and illustrated in Chapter Eight.

Key Points of Chapter Seven

- Even a *Debono Moves* novice can make a big difference to a dog.

- Tiny, gentle movements along a dog's spine may alleviate stiffness.

- The quality of our attention facilitates our dog's improvement.

- Rhythmic movements may bring comfort to a stiff or ailing dog.

- Overusing parts of the body can lead to arthritis and other degenerative changes, creating a vicious cycle which quickly ages a dog. *Debono Moves* can interrupt

---

Method® Practitioner who will address your individual needs. I am based in San Diego County, California, USA, but can travel to work with groups of people. Visit www.DebonoMoves.com for more information or contact me at mary@debonomoves.com. To locate a *Guild Certified Feldenkrais Practitioner*^{cm} in your area, visit www.Feldenkrais.com.

this cycle by helping dogs move in a more balanced way.

- Supporting an area with your hands can reduce strain, promote relaxation, and invite healing.

- Engaging in novel activities helps us feel that time isn't moving so fast.

- To stimulate improvements in functioning, the brain doesn't need big movements. It just needs new ideas.

- Embracing the **Seven Suggestions** can enrich your dog's life – and your own.

- We can all become partners in healing with our dogs.

Chapter Eight: Human Exercises

Please review the "Guidelines for Doing the Exercises" in Chapter One before doing the following exercises.

Human Exercise #1: Deeper Breath, Lighter Hands

Benefits: This exercise can help you discover a more efficient way to breathe, which may improve stamina and reduce stress. This exercise also guides you to lighter, more refined use of your hands, freeing you of unnecessary tension and improving your ability to do *Debono Moves* to help your dog.

This exercise is referred to in Chapter Two.

Listen to the audio recording of this exercise by going to www.debonomoves.com/dog-book and typing in the password *free.*

1. Lie on your back. For comfort, you can put a pillow or rolled-up blanket under your knees and a folded towel under your head. Let your arms lie comfortably at your sides.

2. Without changing anything, simply notice your breathing. What parts of you move as you breathe? Does your abdomen rise when you inhale or when you exhale? When does your chest rise? When does it fall?

3. Place one hand on your lower abdomen and the other on your chest. Let your hands sense the movement in your chest and abdomen as you breathe.

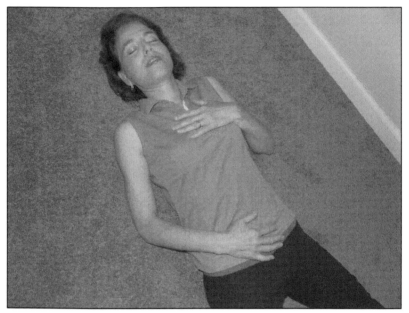

Place one hand on your abdomen and the other on your chest.

4. As you inhale, gently expand your abdomen. At the same time, flatten your chest. When you exhale, flatten your abdomen and expand your chest. Make these movements distinct, but also gentle and light. Do not strain. Breathe like this for a couple of minutes, then rest. Breathe naturally.

5. Without doing anything special, notice how you are breathing now. Is your abdomen expanding when you inhale or when you exhale? What is happening in your chest?

6. Let your arms rest at your sides. Is it more comfortable to have the palms of your hands facing up or down? Or do you prefer to have your hands resting on the pinky sides? Explore all three ways and notice which one feels the most comfortable.

In the directions that follow, I direct you to start with your right hand. But if it's more comfortable to move your left hand, simply replace "right" with "left" in the following instructions. If it's a strain to keep your legs long, you can put a rolled up blanket under your knees or simply bend your knees and stand your feet on the floor.

7. With your right hand either palm up or resting on its pinky side, begin a slow, gentle movement of bringing your right index finger and right thumb toward each other. Make it a slow, light movement. They don't need to touch, but to simply *move toward each other.* Do that several times, reducing your effort each time. Where can you release unnecessary tension? Does relaxing your eyes and jaws help you make this movement lighter and easier? How does your breathing affect this movement? Pause.

8. Move your right middle finger and thumb toward each other a few times. Again, they don't need to touch. We are looking to improve the ease and quality of the movement, not the size. *When the quality of the movement improves, the movement can get larger without effort or strain.* After several movements, pause.

9. Move your right ring finger and thumb toward each other several times. As always, explore ways to make this movement lighter and easier. Notice where in your body you can eliminate unnecessary tension. Aim for ease and elegance. Pause.

10. Move your right pinky and thumb toward each other several times. Don't forget to move your thumb toward your pinky as well as your pinky toward your thumb. Notice your breathing. Pause.

11. Move the four fingers of your right hand toward your right thumb. As you do so, your hand will have an approximate shape of a bell. Have all four fingers contact the thumb at the same time. It may help to imagine the movement of a jellyfish.

   Think of the *movement originating in the center of your palm*, rather than from the individual fingers. How does this change the movement? Does it become lighter and easier? Can you create a delicate folding of your hand? Are you breathing in a relaxed way?

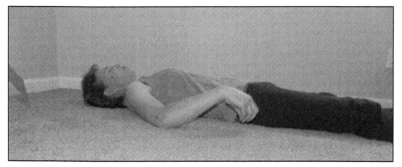

As you move your four fingers toward your thumb, imagine a jellyfish.

   If it's not completely easy for your fingers to touch your thumb, imagine that you have rays of colored light emitting from each fingertip. Direct your movement so that the rays of light will reach your thumb at the same time. Imagine your thumb has a ray of light too.

After several movements, rest.

12. Which hand has more sensation? With your hands still palm down, bring the four fingertips of your right hand toward your right thumb, creating a bell shape again. After a few movements, do the bell-shaped movements with

your left hand. Does one hand move more delicately and accurately? Do you think it would be more pleasant to be touched with your right hand or your left hand?

13. Alternate moving your right and left hands in the bell shape. Feel the movement originate in the center of your palms. Imagine two jellyfish, each one taking a turn at closing and opening. Find a rhythm to this delicate movement. Remember to let each hand open completely before it starts to close again. Can your breathing support these rhythmic movements? After a minute or two, pause and rest.

14. Cross your arms over your lower ribs or abdomen. With your arms hanging comfortably, begin the alternating, rhythmic opening and closing of your hands. Does having your left hand on the right side of your body affect the quality of your movement? Can you imagine that your left hand is *actually* your right hand and vice versa?

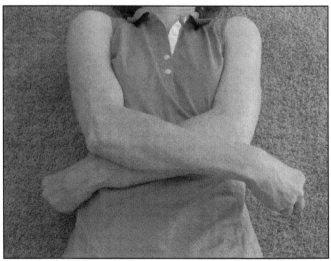

Imagine that your left hand is your right hand and vice versa.

15. Rest with your arms at your sides. How do your arms and hands feel now? In what position are they resting? How does the right hand compare to the left now?

16. Move each individual finger of your left hand toward your left thumb. Do a few movements of each finger and then rest.

17. Place one hand on your chest and the other on your abdomen. Inhale, expanding your abdomen and flattening your chest. Exhale, flattening your abdomen and expanding your chest. Do so gently. Reduce effort throughout yourself. Notice how sensitive your hands feel. How much movement are you aware of now? After a couple of minutes, rest and breathe simply. Let your arms be down at your sides.

18. Notice how you are breathing. How much of you moves as you breathe? How does this compare to how you felt at the start of this exercise? Does your abdomen expand on inhalation now? What happens in your chest? Can you relax more deeply now?

19. When you are ready, slowly roll to your side and sit up. Take some time before you stand up. Slowly walk around, noticing how you feel. If your dog is nearby, gently stroke her. Does your touch have a different quality now?

Human Exercise #2: Improve Your Walking by Lying Down

Benefits: Just as the recumbent Rocky improved his walking, you can too! This relaxing exercise contains movements that occur when you walk. By doing the movements while lying down, you can harness the power of your brain to learn how to walk more easily and efficiently. More comfortable walking reduces wear and tear damage and can help you feel more youthful!

This exercise is referred to in Chapter Two.

Listen to the audio recording of this exercise by going to www.debonomoves.com/dog-book and typing in the password *free*.

1. Lie on your back with your legs long. If it's not comfortable for you to have your legs long, bend both your knees and have your feet flat on the floor, about hip width apart.

2. Notice your contact with the floor. Feel the parts of you that rest against the floor, such as your head, pelvis and heels. Then notice the places that are lifted away from the floor, such as the curve of your neck, the small of your back and the space behind your knees. What other places are lifted up? Does one leg feel longer or wider than the other? Is one foot more turned out?

3. Bend both your knees and stand your feet on the floor, about hip width apart. Place your feet where you don't need to expend effort to keep them in this position. Experiment to find out where that place is. Move your feet a bit away from your pelvis and notice how that feels. Then move them closer to your pelvis. Move your feet apart from each other for a moment and then closer together. Feel how placing your feet most efficiently can reduce your effort. Exploring how you can reduce your effort is an important component of *Debono Moves. Unnecessary effort takes you away from your goals and can lead to fatigue, strain and wear and tear damage.*

4. Open your left knee out to the side. Drop it comfortably toward the floor. If you feel a stretch or strain in your leg, you can prop your knee on a pillow. Keep your right foot standing. Adjust

your position so that it is comfortable for you. Your right foot should be close to the sole of your left foot.

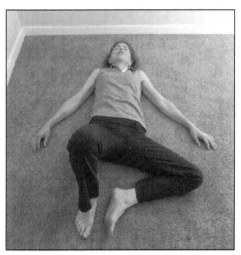

Open your left knee out to the side
and keep your right foot standing.

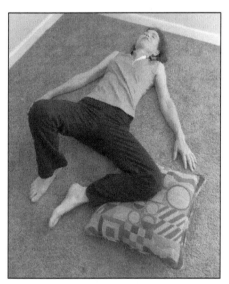

You can prop your knee up with
a pillow for comfort.

5. Press your right foot into the floor so that your right hip comes off the floor a little bit. This doesn't have to be a big movement. Do you press more with your heel or the ball of your foot? Can you feel movement in your spine when you press with your foot? How high up do you feel movement? Press your foot lightly and then release the pressure. Repeat that a few times, making a mental note of how the movement feels. Rest.

6. Put the sole of your right foot *on top* of your left foot. Your left foot is still turned on its side. You can adjust the placement of your feet for comfort and efficiency. As before, press your right foot so that your right hip lifts a little bit. How does this non-habitual movement feel? Do the movement a few times and rest.

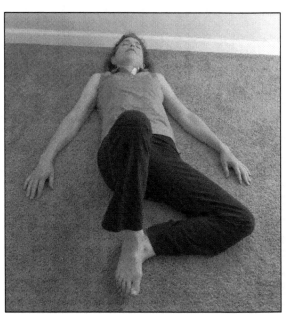

Put your right foot on top of your left foot.
Press with your right foot so that your right
hip lifts a little bit.

7. Move your right foot onto your left ankle and again gently press your right foot a few times. How does this feel? Notice how much your right hip lifts *easily*.

8. Move your right foot higher up your leg so that it rests on your left calf. Press with your right foot a few times and feel how your right hip lifts.

9. Move your right foot higher up your left leg so that it rests below your left knee. Press your right foot a few times so that your right hip lifts.

10. Place your right foot on top of your bent left knee. Press your right foot against your knee a few times.

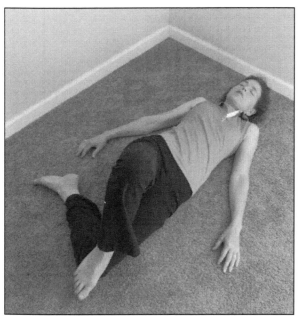

Place your right foot on top of your left knee.

11. Place your right foot on your left thigh and press a few times.

12. If it's easy for you, place your right foot on the floor beyond your left thigh. Press here a few times. How much power do you feel in this position?

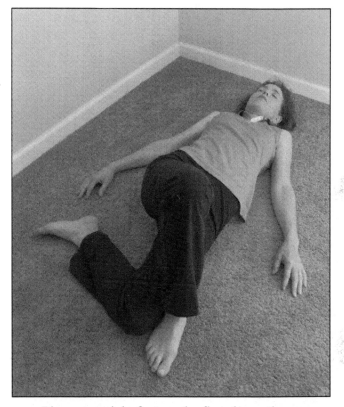

Place your right foot on the floor beyond your left thigh.

13. Place your right foot on the floor next to your left foot. This is the position from Instruction #5. Press the floor with your right foot. How high does your right hip lift now? How far up does the movement travel through your

body? How much of your spine moves? Can you feel your head moving? Is the movement both larger and easier at the same time?

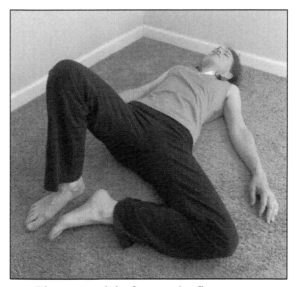

Place your right foot on the floor next to your left foot.

14. Lengthen both of your legs and rest. Feel your contact with the floor and compare it to the beginning of this exercise. Does one leg feel longer or wider than the other? Is one leg more relaxed?

15. Bend your knees and stand your feet. Open your right knee out to the side. Press your left foot against the floor. We'll go through the movements again, this time using your left foot.

16. Press your left foot into the floor so that your left hip comes off the floor a little bit. This doesn't have to be a big movement. Do you press more with your heel or the ball of your foot? Can you feel movement in your spine when you press with your foot? How high up do you feel movement? Press your foot lightly and then release the pressure. Repeat

that a few times, making a mental note of how the movement feels. This side may already be easy, since your brain learned how to do it from the other side. But let's see if you can improve even more!

17. Put the sole of your left foot *on top* of your right foot. Your right foot is still turned on its side. You can adjust the placement of your feet for comfort and efficiency. As before, press your left foot so that your left hip lifts a little bit. How does this non-habitual movement feel? Do the movement a few times and rest.

18. Move your left foot onto your right ankle and again gently press your left foot a few times. How does this feel? Notice how much your left hip lifts *easily*.

19. Move your left foot higher up your leg so that it rests on your right calf. Press with your left foot a few times and feel how your left hip lifts.

20. Move your left foot higher up your right leg so that it rests below your right knee. Press your left foot a few times so that your left hip lifts.

21. Place your left foot on top of your bent right knee. Press your left foot against your knee a few times.

22. Place your left foot on your right thigh and press a few times.

23. If it's easy for you, place your left foot on the floor beyond your right thigh. Press here a few times. How much power do you feel in this position?

24. Place your left foot on the floor next to your right foot. Press the floor with your left foot. How high does your left hip lift now? How far up does the movement travel through your

body? How much of your spine moves? Can you feel your head moving? Is the movement larger and easier at the same time?

25. Lengthen both of your legs and rest. Feel your contact with the floor and compare it to the beginning of this exercise. How do your legs compare to each other now?

26. Slowly roll to your side and walk around. Is there a difference in the quality and ease of your walking?

Human Exercise #3: Easier Sitting

Benefits: Like our canine friends Cassie and Otis, many humans restrict the movement of their spine, which can lead to stiffness and injury. This exercise can help you sit in a way that not only feels better, but can improve the health of your spine.

Sitting more comfortably will also enable you to do *Debono Moves* more easily and effectively with your dog.

This exercise is referred to in Chapter Three.

Listen to the audio recording of this exercise by going to www.debonomoves.com/dog-book and typing in the password *free*.

For the sitting lessons, please sit on a chair that has a flat, firm seat. If there is padding on the chair seat, it should be minimal. You don't want to sink into the chair, so an armchair, sofa or bed is not recommended for these exercises. The chair should be tall enough so that your hips are at least as high as your knees.

1. Please sit comfortably on your chair. How are you breathing? Notice how your weight is distributed. Do you

have more pressure on one hip compared to the other? Are you leaning to one side? Is your back straight or rounded? Are your feet flat on the floor or tucked underneath your chair? How far apart are your feet? Does sitting up feel like an effort? Look in front of you and note what you see on the horizon.

2. Slide forward so that you are sitting towards the front of your chair, with your feet flat on the ground. Place your feet a comfortable distance from each other, about hip width apart. Let your arms rest in your lap. Look up towards the ceiling once or twice, only moving as far as is entirely easy and comfortable. Mentally mark the spot, either on the ceiling or the wall in front of you that your eyes arrived at. Rest.

3. Put the palm of one hand against your lower back. If it's not comfortable to put your palm against the small of your back, place the back of your hand there. Lean forward from your hips, keeping your back straight. Your lower back should stay fairly straight as you do this, getting neither convex nor concave. This movement is referred to as *bending at the hip joints*. Only go as far as it is comfortable and easy. Do this a few times and then rest.

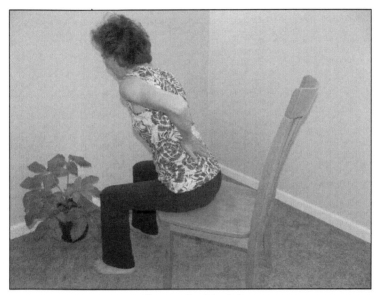

Bending at the hip joints.

4. Put the palm of one hand against your lower back again. This time, gently round your back as if you were slouching. Can you feel how your lower back pushes out against your hand as your pelvis tilts backward? Do you feel how you sit on the back of your seat bones? This movement is referred to as rounding, or *flexing*, your spine.

Put your hands on "hip bones" so that you can feel how your pelvis moves backward when you round your back.

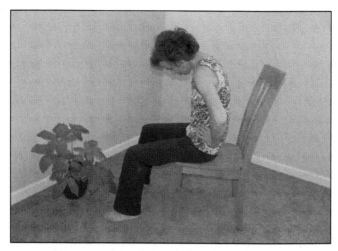

The top of your pelvis moves backward when you round your back.

Do this rounding movement a few times. Rounding your spine is very different than bending from the hip joints. Can you feel the difference? Round your spine a few times and then rest. If you'd like to make sure that you can tell the difference between rounding your back and bending from the hip joints, repeat Instruction #3. Notice that the top of your pelvis moves *forward* (not backward) when you bend from your hip joints. And your back stays straight.

5. Place your hand on your lower back again. Gently push out your belly so that your lower back arches, becoming more concave. Can you feel how your pelvis tilts forward and your weight shifts onto the front of your seat bones? If you put a hand on each "hip bone," you can feel your pelvis tilting forward. Do this arching movement a few times, making it lighter and easier each time. Rest.

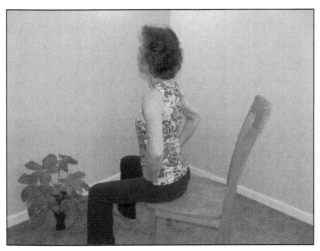

The top of your pelvis moves forward when you arch your back.

6. Put your other hand on your lower back. Alternate rounding and arching your back. What is your head doing? Let your chin drop down toward your chest as you round your back. Then let your chin lift up as you arch your back. Think of all the vertebrae of your spine participating in these movements. Try exhaling as you round your back and inhaling as you arch. Then try the opposite. Which is easier? Does exhaling when you round your back help you soften your chest and make bending your spine easier? Do the movements several times, then rest.

7. Let your hands hang down between your thighs. Repeat the rounding and arching movements as in the previous instruction. This time, though, rotate your arms inward as you round your back and outward as you arch your back. Let your knees move together as your arms rotate inward. Let your knees open as your arms rotate outward. Think of yourself as a flower closing in on itself as you round and opening up to the sunlight as you arch your back and gently look up. Move slowly and pleasurably several times. Rest.

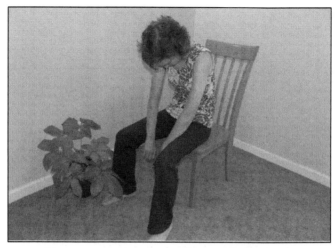

Rotate your arms *inward* as you *round* your back. Your knees will come closer together.

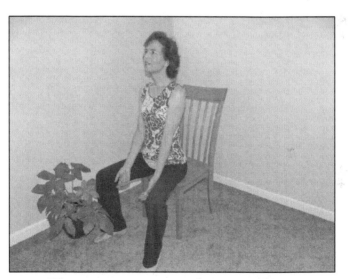

Rotate your arms *outward* as you *arch* your back. Your knees will open out.

8. With your hands hanging down, round and arch your back as in the previous instruction, but this time rotate your arms *outward* as you *round* your back and *inward* as you

arch your back. Does this feel more challenging? Easier? Move slowly and pleasurably several times. Now do the opposite, rotating your arms inward as you round your back and outward as you arch your back. How does that compare? Explore this movement a couple of times and then rest.

9. With your hands resting on your thighs, round and arch your back. You don't need to do anything special with your arms this time. Instead, we'll explore non-habitual movements of your eyes. Please direct your *eyes up toward your eyebrows* as you round your back. Your chin will still go toward your chest, but your *eyes* will look up. When you arch your back and lift your chin, *direct your eyes down,* toward your cheekbones. Do these movements slowly several times.

   Make the movements easier and lighter. The size of the movements does not matter. As always, we are looking to improve the *quality* of the movements. After several movements, return to having your eyes lead the movement, so that you are looking down as you round your back and up when you arch. Is the movement easier and lighter now? What has changed? Explore the movement once or twice more and then rest.

10. Notice how you are sitting on your chair now. Do you feel your seat bones more clearly? Look straight ahead and notice what you see. Are you looking at a different spot in front of you? If so, your head is probably held in a different position than before. Are you sitting more erect without effort? Can you feel how your bones can support you in sitting? Look up. Are you seeing a different spot than when you first started this exercise?

11. Slowly stand up. Gently round and arch your back in standing, then walk around. Notice what feels different.

Variations

Note: Sitting on a rolled-up blanket or large pillow may make it easier for you to sit on the floor, as it can ease strain on the hips.

- Instead of sitting in a chair, do the movements while sitting cross-legged on the floor. After a few movements, change which leg is crossed in front. Are the movements easier when a particular leg is in front?

- Sit on the floor with your legs spread comfortably in front of you. How do the movements feel in this position?

- Sit on the floor and put the soles of your feet together. Can you do the movements easily in this position?

Human Exercise #4: Lengthen Your Hamstrings Without Stretching

Benefits: Like Otis the Boxer, many people suffer from tight hamstrings. This exercise will help you feel the relationship between your hamstrings and your back. By learning to move your spine freely, you can improve your flexibility and naturally lengthen your hamstrings.

This exercise is referred to in Chapter Three.

Listen to the audio recording of this exercise by going to www.debonomoves.com/dog-book and typing in the password *free*.

1. Stand with your feet about hip width apart. Gently bend down, letting your hands move toward your feet. It's important that you do not stretch or force the movement in any way. *Simply notice how far you reach without any*

stretching or straining whatsoever. Then return to standing upright.

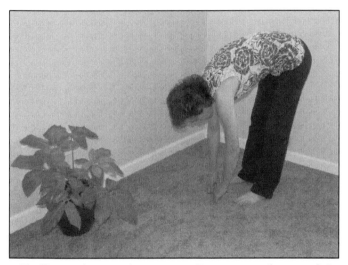

Easily reach toward your toes. Do not stretch or strain!

2. Bend your knees slightly. Put your right hand on your thigh, just above your right knee. Put your left hand just above your left knee. Let the weight of your upper body rest on your hands. Pulling your belly inward, gently round your back and look down. Then, pushing your belly out, gently arch your back, lift your head and look up. Stick your tail out! Do these movements several times, alternating between rounding and arching your back.

If it's uncomfortable for you to lean on your bent knees, do not continue. Instead, refer to the variation following this list of directions.

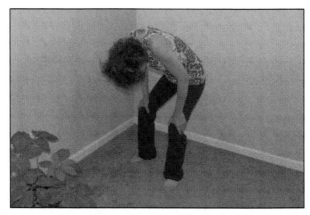

Round your back and look down.

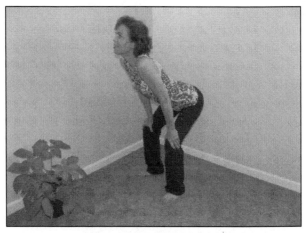

Arch your back and look up.

As you alternately round and arch your back, put your attention on your entire spine. Think of all the vertebrae of your spine participating in these movements. Many of us get into habits of overusing some parts of our spine and underusing others. Let these movements be an opportunity for you to "wake up" the parts of your spine that have been underutilized, while you let the overworked parts do only their fair share. Notice what it feels like when the movement is distributed appropriately throughout your spine. Does the movement get easier and lighter?

3.   Return to standing and bend forward, allowing your hands to go down toward your feet as in the first instruction. Do you notice any change? Rest for a moment.

4.   Stand with your feet spread and your knees slightly bent. Lean with both hands just above your left knee. Like before, slowly and gently round and arch your back. As you round your back, look down and gently pull your belly in. As you arch your back, look up and let your belly come forward. It's important that you not hold in your abdominal muscles. Do these alternating move-ments several times. Then stand and rest for a moment. Notice how you are standing.

5.   Stand with both feet spread about hip width. Lean both your hands on your right thigh, just above the knee. Again, gently round and arch your back as you did previously. Is it different than when you leaned on your left leg? After a few movements, stand and rest.

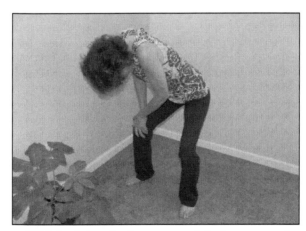

With both hands above your right knee, round your back and look down.

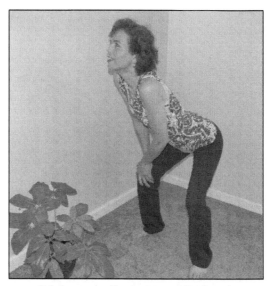

Stick your tail out as you look up!

6. Stand with your feet spread as before and bend down
   toward your feet, allowing your arms to hang. Do you
   bend more easily? Are your hands closer to your toes?

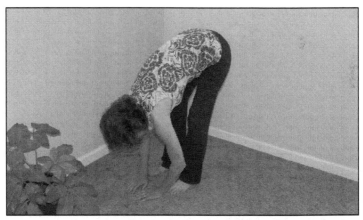

Can you more *easily* reach toward your toes now?

Did you notice that you improved your flexibility without stretching or straining? By doing the movements with attention, your brain learned how to let go of tight leg and back muscles and produce easier, more comfortable movement.

Variation

1. Stand with your feet about hip width apart. Gently bend down, letting your hands move toward your feet. It's important that you do not stretch or force the movement in any way. *Just notice how far you reach without any stretching or straining whatsoever.* Then return to standing upright.

2. **Place your hands on a table or a solid chair**. Drop your weight into your hands. Pulling your belly inward, gently round your back and look down. Then, pushing your belly out, gently arch your back, lift your head and look up. Stick your tail out! Do these movements several times, alternating between rounding and arching your back.

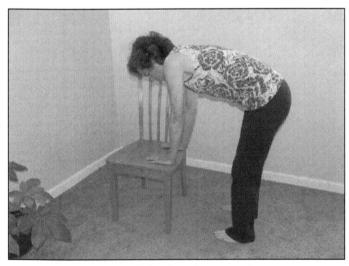

Let your weight drop into your hands.

As you alternately round and arch your back, put your attention on your entire spine. Think of all the vertebrae of your spine participating in these movements. Many of us get into habits of overusing some parts of our spine and underusing others. Let these movements be an opportunity for you to "wake up" the parts of your spine that have been underutilized, while you let the overworked parts do only their fair share. Notice what it feels like when the movement is distributed appropriately throughout your spine. Does the movement get easier and lighter?

3.   Return to standing and bend forward, allowing your hands to go down toward your feet as in the first instruction. Do you notice any change? Rest for a moment.

4.   Put your hands on the table or chair again. Alternately round and arch your back, but this time *reverse the habitual movement of your eyes.* When you round your back and your chin drops toward your chest, raise your eyes so that you are looking toward your eyebrows. Pay attention that your face still drops downward, though.

When you arch your back and your chin lifts away from your chest, direct your eyes to look down toward your cheekbones. Can you still keep a feeling of ease and lightness while making these non-habitual movements with your eyes?

5.   Return to moving your eyes in the habitual way (i.e., look down when you round your back and look up when you arch your back). Do your neck and back move more freely now? Round and arch your back two or three times.

6.   Stand with your feet spread as before and bend down toward your feet, allowing your arms to hang. Do you bend more easily? Are your hands closer to your toes? Did you improve your flexibility without stretching or straining?

Human Exercise #5: Stirring the Soup

Benefits: Many people habitually slump. This exercise can counter that tendency by helping you sit upright effortlessly. It can also improve the mobility of your ribcage, back and pelvis. As we've seen with Nicky, improving the movement of those areas can enhance the flexibility and comfort of the neck and shoulders.

Stirring the Soup will also help you do **Ribcage Circles** with your dog more easily and effectively, helping your dog feel better too!

As with all the exercises, do only what is completely comfortable for you. If you have soreness in your neck, you might want to try the variation that follows these instructions.

This exercise is referred to in Chapter Four.

Listen to the audio recording of this exercise by going to www.debonomoves.com/dog-book and typing in the password *free*.

1. Sit toward the front of a flat-bottomed chair. Have your feet flat on the floor, slightly spread. Feel how your seat bones make contact with the chair. Does one side feel heavier than the other? Does one foot press heavier into the floor? Just notice differences; don't attempt to change them.

2. Cross your right arm over your chest to hold onto your left shoulder with your right hand. Your left hand then goes underneath your right arm and holds onto your right shoulder. *Not everyone can easily hold onto their shoulders, so adjust this position so that it is comfortable for you to maintain. You might need to hold onto your upper arms or elbows.*

3. Letting your chin drop downward, gently round your back so that your weight goes onto the back of your seat bones. Your feet stay quietly on the floor. *If you exhale as you do this movement, your chest will be freer to soften and assist the movement of the spine.* Your elbows will be hanging down.

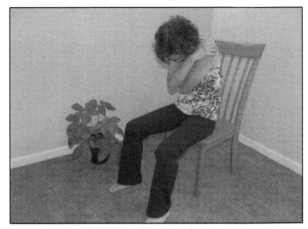

With your arms crossed, round your back
and look down.

4.   Now arch your back, putting your weight onto the front of
      your seat bones. Lift your face and elbows up. Put your
      attention on your entire spine, so that all of it gently
      participates in this arching movement. Think of your elbows
      gently reaching toward the ceiling.

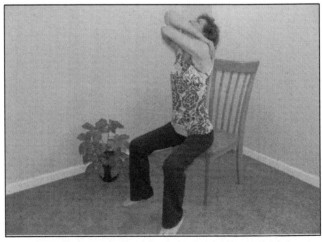

With your arms crossed, arch your back and look up.

5. Alternate these two movements a few times, rounding your back and looking down, and then arching your back and looking up. Go slowly and easily. Move only as far as it's comfortable. Breathe easily. After a few movements, lower your arms and rest. *It's not the size of the movement that is important, but the quality of your attention and the ease you feel.*

6. Cross your arms the other way, with your left arm on top, holding onto the right shoulder. Your right hand will hold onto your left shoulder from below. Look down, rounding your back and then look up, arching your back. Repeat a few times. Does the movement feel different with your arms crossed this way? Lower your arms and rest.

7. Cross your arms with the right arm on top, holding onto the left shoulder. The left hand holds onto the right shoulder from underneath. Let your elbows hang comfortably. Push your right foot into the floor a little bit as you lift the right side of your pelvis off the chair. At the same time, tilt your right ear toward your right shoulder. You'll be bending to your right side. Then straighten back up, sitting on both seat bones and keeping your arms crossed. Repeat a few times and rest.

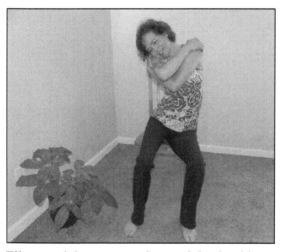

Tilt your right ear toward your right shoulder
as you lift the right side of your pelvis.

8.   Now try it on the left side. Lift your left seat bone and tilt your left ear toward your left shoulder. Repeat a few times and then rest.

9.   Alternate lifting the right side of your pelvis off the chair, then the left side. Do easy, light movements. Lower your arms and rest.

10. Reverse the crossing of your arms and repeat the alternating movements. Let your head gently tilt side-to-side. Lower your arms and rest.

11. Cross your arms with the right arm on top. Hold your elbows straight out in front of you and shift your weight in a circle. I like to pretend that I have a large spoon hanging from my crossed elbows and I'm stirring a big pot of soup. Let your elbows make a big circle. As you "stir the soup," feel how you shift your weight on your pelvis. Feel where it's natural to round your back and shift onto the back of your seat bones. Then feel where you lift one side of your pelvis off the chair, followed by arching your back as your elbows reach out in front of you. Do several circles in each direction, then lower your arms and rest.

*We refer to these circular movements as **Pelvic Circles**. You'll use this movement in several of the **Debono Moves** you'll do with your dog, including Ribcage Circles, Muscle Rolls and Lumbar Circles.*

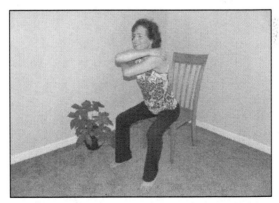

As you "stir the soup," feel how you shift
your weight in a circle.

187

12. Cross your arms the other way and keep stirring the soup! After several circles, lower your arms and rest.

13. Notice how you are sitting in your chair now. How is your weight distributed on your seat bones? How do your feet make contact with the floor? Gently look up and down. Is that easier to do now? Does your whole spine and pelvis help you look up and down now? *This can improve the suppleness of your spine, free up your arms and help reduce your chance of overuse injuries.*

14. Slowly stand up and walk around. Notice your ease of movement.

Variation

This variation can be particularly helpful to those with minor neck soreness. It's also a good way to maintain a happy and comfortable neck, so it's nice to do when you take a computer break. As always, use utmost care and only do what is safe and comfortable for you.

Follow the directions for the exercise above with the following modification. With all the movements, *rest your head completely* on your crossed arms. Even when your back is arching, continue to rest your forehead on your arms. Your elbows will point upward, but your head will remain on your arms and your face will point down.

The same is true when you are shifting your weight in a circle to "stir the soup." Let your head rest heavily on your arms, eliminating any work in your neck.

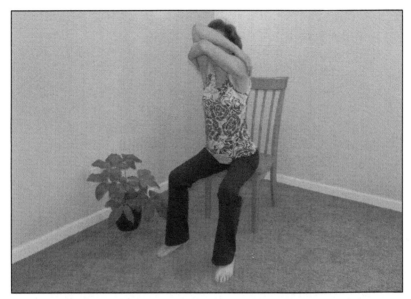

For this variation, let your head rest on your arms even when your back is arching.

Human Exercise #6: Turning Toward a Supple Spine

Benefits: This exercise can help you move more parts of your spine, which helps you turn more easily. It can also improve the movement and comfort of your neck, back and hips.

This exercise is referred to in Chapter Four.

Listen to the audio recording of this exercise by going to www.debonomoves.com/dog-book and typing in the password *free.*

1. Stand with your feet comfortably apart. Turn to look over your right shoulder, then over your left shoulder. Make a mental note of how smooth this turning feels.

2. Lie on your back with your legs long. Notice how your body contacts the floor. How does your right leg compare to your left? Does one leg feel longer or wider? Is one foot more turned out?

How do your shoulders feel? Does one feel higher than the other? Notice how your arms are lying on the floor at your sides. Feel the back of your ribs against the floor. Do you notice differences between your two sides?

Roll your head, *very slowly*, a *tiny* bit from side to side. Does your head roll more easily in one direction? Make sure that you do a very small, slow movement so that you can feel *how* you roll your head. With a large or fast movement, you won't be able to discern subtle, but important, differences.

3. Bend your knees and stand your feet. Cross your right leg completely over the left one so that the back of your right thigh touches the front of your left thigh. You can shift your left foot toward the middle to help you maintain your balance. Slowly, do a small movement of tilting your knees to the right and then back to the middle.

Make this movement small and easy. Move just enough so that you can feel your weight shift on your left foot. Repeat this movement many times, each time going a little farther to the right, as long as it stays easy and comfortable. Let your head roll to the right as your knees tilt.

As you tilt your knees to the right, push out your belly and arch your back. Does this help you go farther with less effort? To bring your knees back to the middle, pull in your abdomen and flatten your back. After doing this movement several times, pause and rest. You can lengthen your legs if that is comfortable for you.

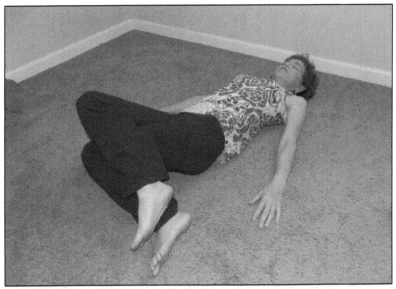

As you tilt your knees to the right, push out your belly and arch your back.

4. Bend your knees. Take a moment to determine the most efficient place to put your feet. Find the place that requires the least amount of effort to hold your knees upright.

    Bring your arms up toward the ceiling. Put your palms together and keep your elbows straight. With your arms in this triangle, tilt your arms to the left and back to the middle. Start with very small movements, letting the movement get a bit larger each time. Move only within your range of comfort and ease.

    Can you feel your right shoulder sliding over your ribs? Let your head roll to the left as your arms tilt to the left. Breathe in an easy, comfortable way. Do the movement many times, then lower your arms and rest.

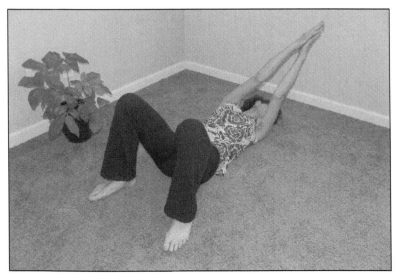

Keep your palms together and your elbows straight as you tilt your arms.

5. With your arms by your side, cross your right leg over your left leg, as you did earlier. Tilt your knees to the right a few times. Does this feel different now? Do you tilt your legs farther now? Is the movement easier? Just do a few movements, then uncross your legs and rest.

    Many people find that they improve their ability to tilt their legs to the side after tilting their arms in the opposite direction. When you tilt your crossed legs, you are rotating the lower part of your spine. When you tilt your arms in the opposite direction, the upper part of your spine rotates in the opposite direction. It's a bit like wringing out a dishrag! You turn one end in one direction and the other end in the opposite direction. Moving your spine in this way helps you recruit all the different parts of your back, even the ones you habitually "tune out." It's a wonderful way to enhance the awareness and mobility of your spine.

6. Notice how you contact the floor now. Do parts press either heavier or lighter against the floor compared to when you started the exercise? How do your legs feel? Have your shoulders changed? Roll your head gently from side to side and notice any changes. Rest.

7. Bend your knees and stand your feet. Cross your left leg completely over your right one so that the back of your left thigh touches the front of your right thigh. You can shift your right foot toward the middle to help you maintain your balance. Slowly, do a small movement of tilting your knees to the left and then back to the middle.

    Make this movement small and easy. Move just enough so that you can feel your weight shift on your right foot. Repeat this movement many times, each time going a little farther to the left, as long as it stays easy and comfortable. Let your head roll to the left as your knees tilt.

    As you tilt your knees to the left, push out your belly and arch your back. Does this help you go farther with less effort? To bring your knees back to the middle, pull in your abdomen and flatten your back. After doing this movement several times, pause and rest. You can lengthen your legs if that is comfortable for you.

8. Bend your knees. Take a moment to determine the most efficient place to put your feet. Find the place that requires the least amount of effort to hold your knees upright.

    Bring your arms up toward the ceiling. Put your palms together and keep your elbows straight. With your arms in this triangle, tilt your arms to the right and back to the middle. Start with very small movements, letting the movement get a bit larger each time. Move only within your range of comfort and ease.

Can you feel your left shoulder sliding over your ribs? Let your head roll to the right as your arms tilt to the right. Breathe in an easy, comfortable way. Do the movement many times, then lower your arms and rest.

9.   With your arms by your side, cross your left leg over your right leg, as you did earlier. Tilt your knees to the left a few times. Does this feel different now? Do you tilt your legs farther now? Is the movement easier? Just do a few movements, then uncross your legs and rest.

10. Notice how you contact the floor now. Do parts press either heavier or lighter against the floor compared to when you started the exercise? How do your legs feel? Have your shoulders changed? Roll your head gently from side to side and notice any changes. Rest.

11. Bend your knees and stand your feet. Bring your arms up toward the ceiling. Put your palms together and keep your elbows straight. With your arms in this triangle, tilt your arms to the right and then to the left. Let your head roll as you tilt your arms from side to side. Move only within your range of comfort and ease.

Breathe in an easy, comfortable way. Do the movement many times, then lower your arms and rest.

12. Bring your arms up to the ceiling and make that triangle again. Tilt your arms from side to side, but this time roll your head in the direction opposite direction from your arms. As your arms tilt to the right, gently roll your head to the left. As you tilt your arms to the left, delicately roll your head to the right. Can you make this a simple, easy movement? Do it many times. As always, rest whenever you need to.

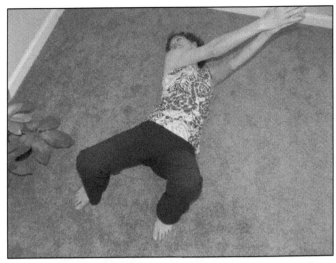

As you tilt your arms to the left, roll your head to the right, and vice versa.

13. As you continue to roll your head opposite to the direction of your tilting arms, move your eyes opposite the direction of your head. In other words, as you tilt your arms to the right, your face will turn to the left, but your eyes will look to the right. As you tilt your arms to the left, your face will turn to the right, and your eyes will look to the left. Go very slowly and just do small movements. Remember to keep your elbows straight and your palms together. Make sure to keep breathing!

    Do several movements, making each movement a bit easier and smoother each time. Return hands, face and eyes to the middle at the same time. This can help you learn how to coordinate your movements more smoothly. Do this movement several times, then pause.

14. With your arms held in the triangle, tilt your arms, face and eyes in the same direction. Go from left to right many times. Do you go easier and farther now? What

has changed?   Do a few movements, then lower your arms and rest.

15.   Roll your head slowly from side to side. How does it feel compared to when you started this exercise? Does your head roll more smoothly and evenly? Has your contact with the floor changed?

16.   Slowly roll to your side and come to sitting. Slowly and smoothly stand up. Turn to look over your right shoulder and then your left shoulder. Has your ability to turn improved? Does it feel easier and smoother? Slowly walk around and notice how your hips feel. Enjoy a feeling of freedom as you go about your day!

Human Exercise #7: Hip and Shoulder Circles

Benefits: This exercise can help you enjoy freer movement in your pelvis and shoulders, while it facilitates more balanced, coordinated movement throughout your whole body.

It can also improve your ability to do **Hip and Shoulder Circles** with your dog so you can help your canine companion move more freely too!

This exercise is referred to in Chapter Five.

Listen to the audio recording of this exercise by going to www.debonomoves.com/dog-book and typing in the password *free*.

1.   Lie on your back with your legs long. Notice your contact with the floor. Feel how your arms and legs are lying. Roll your head gently from side to side.

2.   Lie on your right side. Put some folded towels or a small pillow under your head for comfort. Bend your knees up so that they are resting one on top of the other. Have your left arm draped along your side, with your hand

somewhere near your left hip. Adjust your position for comfort.

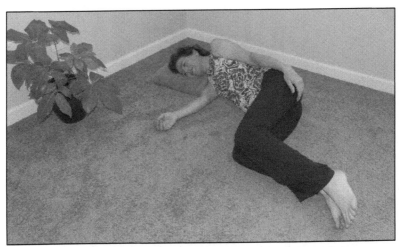

Bend your knees on top of each other and have your left arm along your side.

3. Do a very small movement of bringing your left shoulder a bit forward and then back to its starting place. How can you make this movement easier, lighter, and simpler? Do the movement many times and then rest on your side.

4. Move your left shoulder backward a small amount and then return to its starting place. Do that movement many times, again exploring ways to make the movement smoother and more comfortable. Rest on your side.

5. Take your shoulder a little forward, then a little backward. Go forward and backward many times. Which direction is easier? Are you breathing in a relaxed way? Pause and rest on your side.

6. Gently bring your left shoulder up toward your left ear and then return to neutral. Do that many times. How lightly and easily can you do this movement? Can you

reduce tension in your jaw, throat and neck? Can you smile and breathe? Pause and rest.

7. Drop your shoulder downward toward your hip several times. Is this easier or more challenging than bringing your shoulder up? Make it easy and light. Pause and rest.

8. Alternate taking your left shoulder up toward your ear and then dropping it downward. Do that movement many times. Can both directions feel easy? Pause and rest.

9. You've taken your shoulder in four directions. If you did them one after another, you could make a circle. Let's try that! Lift your left shoulder up toward your ear, then take it forward, then downward and then backward. Do you feel how that makes a circle?

    Do many circles, exploring how you can make them lightly and smoothly. Are there places on your circle that are not round? Can you smooth them out? Does breathing in a relaxed way help? Reduce tension in your eyes, mouth and hands. Where else can you let go of unnecessary effort?

    Do several circles in each direction. Is one direction easier than the other? Can they both feel easy and free?

    Pause and rest on your back. You won't need as much support under your head when you are on your back. Adjust it as needed.

10. Lie on your right side again. Have your knees bent and resting one on top of the other. You can rest your left hand on the floor in front of you.

    Move your left "hip" up toward your head. (Actually, it is the top of the pelvis that you are bringing toward your head, but it is commonly referred to as the "hip", so that is the term we will use in this exercise.)

How do you make this *small, subtle* movement happen? Make sure that you are not lifting your left foot as you do this. Do you feel the *right side of your waist pressing into the floor* as you lift your left hip up toward your head? Do it many times, then pause.

11. Move your left hip downward several times. Is this direction easier or more challenging? Can you feel how to *lift the right side of your waist* to make this movement? Pause after several movements.

12. Alternate taking your left hip up and down many times. Each time, find a way to make the movement lighter and smoother. Feel what is happening in the right side of your waist. These are small, subtle movements. Remember to breathe. Pause.

13. Take your left hip forward a small amount. Do that many times. Your left knee will slide forward, but don't lift your left foot. Make it light and easy. Pause.

14. Take your left hip backward many times. Your left knee will slide backward. Is it easier to take your hip forward or backward? Pause.

15. Alternate between taking your left hip forward and backward a number of times. Pause and rest.

16. Just like you did with your shoulder, you've taken your hip in four directions. Let's piece them together to make a circle. Take your left hip up toward your head, forward, downward and backward. How smooth can you make this circle? Make several circles in each direction, exploring how to make them easier and more fluid. Is one direction easier than the other? Pause and rest on your back.

17. Lie on your right side again. Adjust your head support as needed and bend your knees on top of each other. Drape your left arm along your side.

    Let's explore simultaneously moving your left shoulder and left hip. Take your shoulder downward as you bring your hip up at the same time. Your shoulder and hip will be coming closer together. Can you feel how you are shortening your left side while lengthening your right side? Your left ribs are getting closer together and your right ribs are getting farther apart. Can this movement feel effortless?

    Make this movement many times. Once you've gotten the hang of it, make it lighter and quicker. Don't hurry, just do it faster. Find an effortless rhythm. After many movements, rest on your side.

18. Now let's do the opposite movement. Take your left shoulder up as you take your left hip down. Your shoulder and hip will be moving apart. Feel how you are lengthening on your left side and shortening on your right side.

    Once you've gotten the hang of it, make it lighter and quicker. Find an effortless rhythm. After many movements, rest on your side.

19. Take your shoulder forward and your hip backward. Do that movement many times, making it lighter and smoother each time. Pause.

20. Take your shoulder backward and your hip forward. Is this easier or more challenging? How can you make it simple? Pause after several movements.

21. Alternate taking your shoulder and hip forward and backward. After a few movements, move lightly and quickly. Find an effortless rhythm to this movement. Pause and rest on your side.

22. Now make circles with your left shoulder and left hip simultaneously. You may want to think it through first. Can you breathe in a relaxed way while you coordinate these movements? Which direction did you try first? Do several circles in each direction.

    As always, discover how to make the movements more comfortable. Let go of any tension and discard the habit of straining. Smile! Pause after several movements.

23. Can you imagine doing opposing circles with your shoulder and hip? *Opposing circles* mean that you are making circles in one direction (e.g., clockwise) with your shoulder and circles in the opposite direction (e.g., counterclockwise) with your hip. Even if it doesn't seem possible, *imagine* doing these non-habitual movements. *There's value in your brain mulling over novel movement puzzles.* Can you breathe and smile while imaging something challenging?

    It's helpful to have a friend put her hands on your shoulder and hip and very gently move them in opposing circles. Your brain will sense this novel movement and gain benefits from it. See **Hip and Shoulder Circles** *for your dog in Chapter Five for more information.*

24. Return to doing the hip and shoulder circles in the same direction. Have your circles gotten lighter and easier? Can you feel more movement in your waist? What else has changed? Pause and rest on your back.

25. Notice your contact with the floor. What has changed? How do your shoulders compare to each other? How do your legs feel? Slowly roll your head from side to side. Rest. Can you sense yourself more clearly now? Is more of your body touching the floor?

26. Lie on your left side. Put some folded towels or a small pillow under your head for comfort. Bend your knees up so that they are resting one on top of the other. Have your right arm draped along your side, with your hand somewhere near your right hip. Adjust your position for comfort.

27. Now that your brain has learned how to make the movements easier on your left side, you can improve your right side in a shorter amount of time. You may find that you only need to do a few movements to create a big change.

    Do a small movement of bringing your right shoulder a bit forward and then back to its starting place. How can you make this movement easier, lighter, and simpler? Rest on your side.

28. Move your right shoulder backward a small amount and then return to its starting place. Explore ways to make the movement smoother and more comfortable. Rest on your side.

29. Now take your shoulder a little forward, then a little backward. Go forward and backward many times. Is it easier for you to go backward or forward? Are you breathing as you do this movement? Pause and rest on your side.

30. Gently bring your right shoulder up toward your right ear and then return to neutral. How lightly and easily can you do this movement? Can you reduce unnecessary tension in your jaw, throat and neck? Can you smile and breathe? Pause and rest.

31. Drop your right shoulder downward several times. Is this easier or more challenging than bringing your shoulder up? Make it easy and light. Pause and rest.

32. Take your right shoulder up toward your ear and then downward. Can both directions feel easy? Pause and rest.

33. Take your right shoulder in a circle. Lift your right shoulder up toward your ear, then take it forward, then downward and then backward.

    Explore how you can make these circles lightly and smoothly. Are there places on your circle that are not round? Can you smooth them out? Does breathing in a relaxed way help? Reduce tension in your eyes, mouth and hands. Where else can you let go of unnecessary work?

    Do several circles in each direction. Is one direction easier than the other? Can they both feel easy and free?

    Pause and rest on your back. You won't need as much support under your head when you are on your back. Adjust it as needed.

34. Lie on your left side again. Have your knees bent and resting one on top of the other. You can rest your right hand on the floor in front of you.

    Move your right hip up toward your head. How do you make this small, subtle movement happen? Do you feel the left side of your waist pressing into the floor? Make sure that you are not lifting your right foot. Reduce any unnecessary work, as it will only interfere with your freedom of movement. Pause.

35. Move your right hip downward. Is that easier or more challenging? Can you feel how you have to lift the left side of your waist to make this movement? Pause.

36. Alternate taking your right hip up and down a few times. Each time, find a way to make the movement lighter and smoother. Breathe! Pause.

37. Take your right hip forward a small amount. Your right knee will slide forward, but don't lift your right foot. Make it light and easy. Pause.

38. Take your right hip backward many times. Which is easier, taking your hip forward or backward? Pause.

39. Alternate taking your right hip forward and backward a number of times. Pause and rest.

40. Now take your right hip in a circle. Move your hip up toward your head, forward, downward, and then backward. How smooth can you make this circle? Make several circles in each direction, exploring how to make them easier and more fluid. Is one direction easier than the other? Pause and rest on your back.

41. Lie on your left side again. Adjust your head support as needed and bend your knees on top of each other. Drape your right arm along your side.

   Let's explore simultaneously moving your right shoulder and right hip. Take your shoulder downward as you bring your hip up at the same time. Your shoulder and hip will be coming closer together. Can you feel how you are shortening your right side while lengthening your left side? Your right ribs are getting closer together and your left ribs are getting farther apart. Can you make this movement feel effortless?

   Make this movement many times. Once you've gotten the hang of it, make it lighter and quicker. Don't hurry, just do it faster. Find an effortless rhythm. After many movements, rest on your side.

42. Now let's do the opposite movement. Take your shoulder up as you take your hip down. Your shoulder and hip will be moving apart. Feel how you are lengthening on your right side and shortening on your left side.

   Once you've gotten the hang of it, make it lighter and quicker. Find an effortless rhythm. After many movements, rest on your side.

204

Take your shoulder forward and your hip backward. Do that movement many times, making it lighter and smoother each time. Pause.

43. Take your shoulder backward and your hip forward. Is this easier or more challenging? How can you make it simple? Pause after several movements.

44. Alternate taking your shoulder and hip forward and backward. After a few movements, move lightly and quickly. Find an effortless rhythm to this movement. Pause and rest on your side.

45. Now make circles with your right shoulder and right hip simultaneously. You may want to think it through first. Can you breathe in a relaxed way while you coordinate these movements? Which direction did you try first? Do several circles in each direction.

    As always, discover how to make the movements more comfortable. Let go of any tension and discard the habit of straining. Smile! Pause after several movements.

46. Can you imagine doing opposing circles with your shoulder and hip? Even if it doesn't seem possible, *imagine* doing these non-habitual movements. Can you breathe and smile while imaging something challenging?

    It's helpful to have a friend put her hands on your shoulder and hip and very gently move them in opposing circles. Your brain will sense this novel movement and gain benefits from it. See **Hip and Shoulder Circles** *for your dog in Chapter Five for more information.*

47. Return to doing the hip and shoulder circles in the same direction. Have your circles gotten lighter and easier? Can you feel more movement in your waist? What else has changed? Pause and rest on your back.

48. Notice your contact with the floor. What has changed? How do your shoulders compare to each other? How do your legs feel? Slowly roll your head from side to side. Rest. Can you sense yourself more clearly now? Is more of your body touching the floor?

49. Slowly roll to your side and sit up. Stand up and notice how you feel. Have your shoulders dropped down? Walk around and notice how your arms and legs are swinging. Take a stroll and notice your improvements.

Variations

- To reduce stress and keep shoulder tension at bay, you can do gentle shoulder circles while sitting at your desk or even standing in line at the store. Begin with the individual movements of taking your shoulder forward, backward, upward and downward. Piece these movements together to make a circle just like you did in the above exercise.

- While sitting or standing, do the shoulder movements while looking straight ahead, turning your head toward the shoulder that is moving or turning your head away from the moving shoulder. Try it each way and notice any differences.

- What is it like to move both shoulders at the same time? Are you moving them in identical circles? Can you move one shoulder clockwise and the other counterclockwise? Which way feels more interesting? Make all the movements easy and gentle.

Mindlessly moving your shoulders in circles won't produce the learning that attentive moving does. Take the time to sense and feel how to move more comfortably and freely and you will reap big dividends in mind and body!

Human Exercise #8: Making Time for Freer Hips

Benefits: Many people complain of sore or tight hips. By refining the movement of your pelvis, this exercise can help release restrictions around your hip joints and lower back, leading to happier hips.

This exercise is referred to in Chapter Six.

Listen to the audio recording of this exercise by going to www.debonomoves.com/dog-book and typing in the password *free*.

1. Lie on your back with your legs long. Check to see if you need a folded towel or small pillow under your head. Notice your contact with the floor. How much space is under your lower back? Can you feel the curve of your neck? Notice how each leg feels. Turn your right leg in and out a few times. Then do the same with your left leg. Roll your head a little from side to side.

2. Bend your knees so that your feet are standing. Take a moment to find the most efficient place to put your feet.
   Flatten your lower back by gently pressing the floor with your feet. Make this a small, light movement. Don't hold the position, simply flatten your back and then release it. Feel how the top of your pelvis (your "hip bones") moves toward your head. You can put your hands on your "hips" to feel this more clearly.
   Do the movement many times, making it simpler and easier each time. Notice how you are breathing. Release any unnecessary tension. Pause.

3. Now do the opposite movement. Arch your lower back so that it moves away from the floor. You'll create more space between your lower back and the floor. Feel how

the top of your pelvis moves down toward your feet. You can put your hands on your "hips" to feel this more clearly.

Is arching your back away from the floor easier than flattening it? Or is flattening your back easier to do? Pause after several movements.

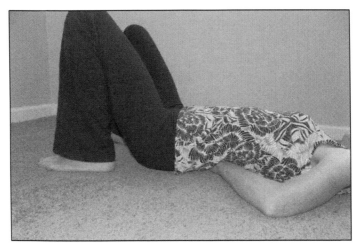

I use my hand to feel the arch I created between my back and the floor.

4. Alternate between arching your back away from the floor and flattening it against the floor. Remember to push against the floor with your feet to flatten your back. This allows you to keep your abdomen free.

   Do you habitually tighten your abdominal muscles? Chronically tensing your abdominals can lead to restrictions in the back and hips. Let your abdomen be free so that your pelvis and back can move unimpeded.

   Is your head moving? Do you feel your chin going toward and away from your chest? Tighten your chest and abdomen and hold your breath. Now resume the pelvic tilts, where you flatten and arch your back. How does this affect your movement?

Then release any tension in your chest and abdomen and breathe freely. Is your movement freer and easier? Does the movement travel freely up your spine to your head?

Gradually make the movement faster and lighter. Can you do the movements quickly, but without hurrying? Are you breathing? Rest with your legs long. Notice your contact with the floor.

5. Bend your knees and stand your feet. Push your right foot into the floor so that the right side of your pelvis lifts a little away from the floor. Do that movement many times. Explore how the placement of your right foot will affect the ease of lifting your pelvis. Pause.

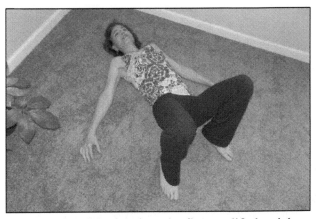

Push your right foot into the floor to lift the right side of your pelvis.

6. Now push your left foot into the floor to lift the left side of your pelvis. Is this side easier or more challenging? What makes it different from lifting your right side? Do the movement many times, always looking to reduce effort. Pause.

7. Alternate between lifting the right and left sides of your pelvis. Make these light, easy movements. After several movements, rest with your legs long. Notice your contact

with the floor. Has it changed since you began this exercise?

8. Bend your knees and stand your feet. You've explored four directions with your pelvis: toward your head (flattening your back), to the left (pushing with your right foot), away from your head (arching your back), and to the right (pushing with your left foot). If you do each of these movements in turn, you will create a circular movement of your pelvis.

   Try it. Flatten your back, then push with your right foot, then arch your back, and then push with your left foot. Can you feel how you just described a circle?

   *We refer to these circular movements as **Pelvic Circles**. You'll find them referenced in parts of the book that describe how to do specific **Debono Moves** with your dog.*

   Imagine that you have a clock painted on the floor beneath your pelvis. When you flatten your back, you touch six o'clock. When you arch your back, you touch 12 o'clock. When you push with your right foot to tilt your pelvis to the left, you touch 9 o'clock. And when you push with your left foot to tilt your pelvis to the right, you contact 3 o'clock.

9. Imagining this clock under your pelvis, make a clockwise circle with your pelvis. Do it slowly, noticing how you can accurately contact all the hours on the clock.

   Take the time to imagine all the hours on your clock. Can you touch 2 o'clock? How about 8 o'clock? How easy is it to touch 10 o'clock? Which hours are easy to touch and which ones are more challenging?

   If you find it difficult to contact certain hours on your clock, make your circles smaller. It's more important to do smaller, round circles, than larger, irregularly-shaped movements.

Take the time to discover how you can coordinate the pushing of each foot to make smooth, even circles. This exercise is valuable because moving your pelvis relative to your hips can release restrictions around your hip joints. I have seen people discover significant improvements in functioning from doing these mindful movements.

As always, rest whenever you need to. When you are ready, make counterclockwise circles. Notice if one direction is easier than the other. Can you make both directions smooth and simple?

Rest with your legs long.

10. Bend your knees and stand your feet. Tilt your pelvis from 12 o'clock to six o'clock by pushing through your feet to flatten your back. Then tilt your pelvis back to 12 o'clock by arching your back. Do this a few times.

    Is the movement traveling more clearly from your feet to your head now? If so, that indicates that you've released restrictions and learned how to move more efficiently.

    Rest with your legs long. Has your contact with the floor changed? Turn each leg in and out a couple of times. How do your legs feel? Roll your head from side to side and notice the freedom in your neck. Perhaps the floor even got more comfortable!

11. Slowly roll to your side and sit up. Then stand up and walk around. Enjoy the newfound freedom in your pelvis, hips and back!

Human Exercise #9: Sitting on a Clock

Benefits: This exercise can help release restrictions around your hip joints and lower back, leading to happier hips and more comfortable sitting and walking.

This exercise can also improve your ability to do the **Debono Moves** that require you to move your pelvis lightly in a circle as you work with your dog.

This exercise is referred to in Chapter Six.

Listen to the audio recording of this exercise by going to www.debonomoves.com/dog-book and typing in the password *free.*

1. Sit toward the front of a flat-bottomed chair. Have your feet flat on the floor, slightly spread. Feel how your seat bones make contact with the chair. Does one side feel heavier than the other? Does one foot press heavier into the floor? Just notice differences; don't attempt to change them.

2. Round your lower back so that your weight goes onto the back of your seat bones. Pull your belly in a little as you do this movement. Your feet stay quietly on the floor. Can you feel how the top of your pelvis moves backward? Put your hands on your "hips" so that you can clearly feel this. Do many movements and then pause.

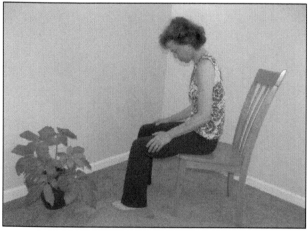

As you round your back, your pelvis tilts backward.

3. Now arch your back, putting your weight onto the front of your seat bones. Push your belly out as you do this. Can you feel how the top of your pelvis tilts forward? Put your hands on your "hips" so that you can feel this. Do many movements and then pause.

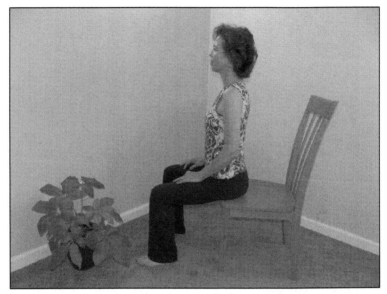

As you arch your back, your pelvis tilts forward.

4. Alternate between rounding your lower back and then arching your lower back. Go slowly and easily. Move only as far as it's comfortable. Breathe easily. After several movements, rest.

5. Return to sitting toward the front of your chair. Push your right foot into the floor a little bit as you lift the right side of your pelvis off the chair. Just lift the right side of your pelvis and put it back down. Don't hold it up. Are you lifting your right heel as you do this? See if you can keep your feet flat on the floor. Repeat a few times and rest.

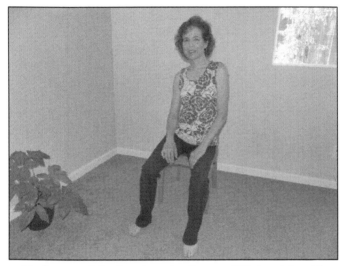

Push your right foot into the floor to lift the right side of your pelvis.

6. Now try it on the left side. Push your left foot into the floor to lift the left side of your pelvis. Do the movement a few times and then rest.

7. Alternate lifting the right side of your pelvis off the chair and then the left side. Do easy, light movements. Reduce your effort. Breathe and smile! After several movements, rest back in your chair.

8. Sit toward the front of your chair again. Imagine that you have a clock painted on the seat of your chair and your pelvis is directly on top of it. Push your belly out and arch your back so that your pelvis tilts downward. You will be contacting 12 o'clock.

9. Pull your belly in and round your back. As your pelvis tilts backward, you'll contact 6 o'clock. Go back and forth between six and 12 o'clock several times. Does your head respond to this movement? Does your chin get closer and

farther away from your chest? Rest after several movements.

10. Push your right foot into the floor to tilt your pelvis to the left. That's 9 o'clock. Then tilt your pelvis to the right to contact 3 o'clock. Go back and forth between 3 o'clock and 9 o'clock several times. Make the movements effortless. Remember to breathe. Rest back in your chair.

11. Sit toward the front of your chair again. Imagining your clock, begin by tilting your pelvis forward to 12 o'clock and then do several clockwise circles. Visualize touching all the hours on your clock. If that doesn't seem possible, make your clock smaller. That means you'll be making smaller circles. Discover how you can make the circles smooth and even.

    We refer to these circular movements as **Pelvic Circles.** *You'll use this movement in several of the* **Debono Moves** *you'll do with your dog, including Ribcage Circles, Muscle Rolls and Lumbar Circles.*

    Hold your breath and tighten your belly. How does that change your ability to make smooth, effortless circles? Can you feel how the habit of holding in your belly can interfere with the health of your spine? Clench your jaws and see how that affects your ability to move. What other places can you restrict?

    Extraneous tension impedes your freedom of movement and creates strain. So let go of any unnecessary tension. Soften your chest and breathe freely. ***Use your belly muscles to round your back, but then immediately release them so that other muscles can work in harmony.*** After many clockwise circles, pause.

12. Make several counterclockwise circles, being mindful to contact every hour on your clock. Aim for smooth, easy circles. Can you feel these circles traveling through your

body? Is your head making circles too? Pause after several movements.

13. Tilt your pelvis forward and back, from 12 o'clock to six o'clock. How has the quality of this movement changed? Notice how your weight is distributed in your chair. Does it feel more even? How are you breathing?

Slowly get up and walk around. Enjoy your free hips and supple spine!

Variations

The brain needs novelty and variety to continue learning and improving.

Instead of doing the exercise in a chair, you might try the following variations:

- Sit cross-legged on the floor. Vary which leg you have crossed in front.

- Sit on the floor with your legs long and spread in front of you.

- Sit on the floor with the soles of your feet together.

- Sit on the floor and then lean back on your elbows and forearms. Put the soles of your feet together.

Human Exercise #10: Better Posture Effortlessly

Benefits: Striving to obtain better posture often leads to strain, fatigue and unhealthy movement. This exercise can help you learn how to be upright without effort, eliminating the rounded back that so often develops from constant sitting and stress.

This exercise also improves the power and use of your back, leading to more coordinated, balanced movement. Discover how you can look, move and feel younger!

This exercise is referred to in Chapter Seven.

Listen to the audio recording of this exercise by going to www.debonomoves.com/dog-book and typing in the password *free.*

1. Lie on your back with your legs long. Notice your contact with the floor. How much space is under your lower back? Can you feel the curve of your neck? Is your head centered over your body? Roll your head a little from side to side. How easy is it to turn your head today?

2. Roll onto your stomach and put your forehead on the floor. Take a moment to make this position comfortable for you. The closer you are to putting your hairline on the floor, the less pressure there will be on your nose.

    Put your hands in a standing position on either side of your head. Your elbows will be pointed toward the ceiling as if you were going to do pushups.

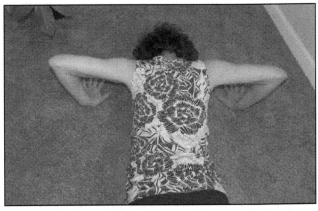

Put your hands in a standing position on either side of your head.

3. Look up at the wall in front of you. Even though your arms are in a pushup position, use your back, not the power of your arms, to look up. How far do you lift your head easily? Don't stretch or strain. Only do what is entirely simple and comfortable. Mentally mark that spot on the wall. Look up once or twice and then rest with your head turned to the side and your arms in a comfortable resting position.

4. Put your forehead on the floor and close your eyes. Gently move your eyes to the right and then back to the middle. Do this movement so gently that you can feel your eyes moving in their sockets. Can you put your attention first on one eye and then the other? Move your eyes to the right many times, making the movements easy and light. Pause.

5. Move your eyes to the left and back to the middle. Do these movements several times. Can you make the movements smooth?

6. Alternate moving your eyes from right to left. Do that many times. Notice if one direction is easier than the other. Which way is more habitual for you to look? Can you make both directions easy? Can you breathe while moving your eyes? Rest with your head to the side.

7. Put your forehead in the middle and close your eyes again. Move your eyes upward, as if you wanted to look at your eyebrows. Return your eyes to the middle. Do this many times. Pause.

8. Move your eyes downward, as if you wanted to look at your cheekbones. Return your eyes to the middle. Do the movement many times. Pause.

9. Alternate between moving your eyes upward and downward. Make the movements smooth and effortless all the way through. Breathe in a relaxed way. Do many movements and then pause.

10. Put your arms in pushup position. Lift your head as if you wanted to look up at the wall in front of you, but look down as you lift your head. Repeat that movement a few times. Lift your head up, but glide your eyes downward. Then, as you begin to lower your head, move your eyes upward. Notice how this reversal of your habit affects your movement. ***When you move in a non-habitual way, something in your brain has to wake up.*** After several movements, pause.

11. With your arms still in pushup position, lift your head to look at the wall in front of you. Let your eyes lead the way so that they are looking up as you lift your head. How high on the wall do you see now? Has something released in your back that lets you lift your head more easily?

    Take a complete rest on your back. Sense what changes occurred from doing those non-habitual movements. Can you feel more of yourself and relax more deeply now?

    Our eyes organize a great deal of our movement, so changing their habitual use can produce substantial improve-ments in our functioning.

12. Roll onto your stomach again. Put your forehead on the floor and your hands resting on either side of your head.

    Slide your forehead down as if you wanted to look at your navel. You'll feel your upper back rounding and lifting toward the ceiling as you do this. Feel how you have to shorten the front of yourself to do this.

    As you do this movement of rounding your upper back, move your eyes upward. As you return your head to the starting position, move your eyes downward. Do this movement many times.

Again, we are reversing your habitual movement. Such novel sensations attract the attention of the brain, leading to improvements in functioning.

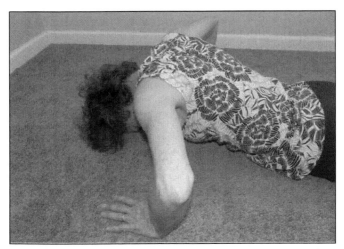

Round your upper back by sliding your head down toward your navel.

13. Put your hands in pushup position. Lift your head and look up at the wall in front of you. How high do you lift your head now? Has something else released which allowed you to use your back more easily and powerfully? Have you suddenly gotten *younger*?

    Roll onto your back and take a nice rest.

14. Lie on your stomach and turn your face to the left. Draw up your left leg so that it is comfortably bent. Your lower leg will still be resting on the mat. Put your right arm down by your side.

    Stand your left hand and turn your fingers outward. Find a place that allows you to push against your left hand in such a way that the force goes up into your left shoulder blade, bringing your shoulder blade closer to your spine. Put your left hand in several different places and push through your hand at each location. Try putting your hand farther away from you and then closer. Which positions make it easier to move your shoulder blade?

Put your left hand far enough away from you that you can feel your shoulder blade slide around. Every few movements, put your hand in a different place, because every new movement will make the movement go through your body in a different path. Many of these new paths will be different from your habits. Be gentle with yourself as you explore these novel movements.

The movements should feel novel, but not uncomfortable. If at any point you find that you not breathing in a relaxed way, you are probably working too hard. In that case, either stop and rest or do the movements more slowly and easily so that you can get back into a learning state.

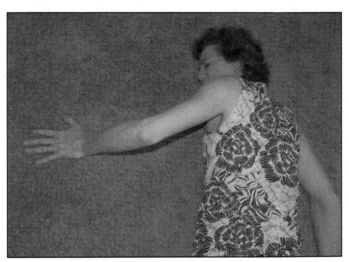

Put your hand in a place that allows you to move your shoulder blade.

15. Slide your left leg down. Stand your left hand closer to your body so that you can produce power when you push through it.

Drag up your left leg as you push against your left hand. Feel how these movements can go together. Do this several times.

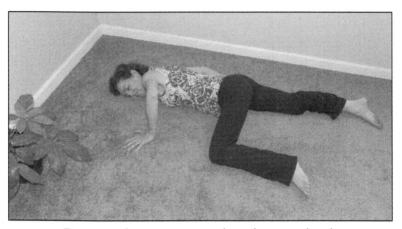

Drag your leg up as you push against your hand.

16. Keep your left leg bent up. Push your left knee away from you and back toward you a few times. Feel the movement in your left hip. Make it simple and light. Feel how this movement engages the deep muscles of your core. After several movements, let your left leg go long.

17. Drag your left leg up again, but this time round your back and bring your head down to look at your knee as your leg comes up. Don't attempt to touch your head to your knee, but simply bring them toward each other. You'll be looking under your arm. Then take them apart, returning your head to the middle and letting your left leg go long. Do that movement several times.

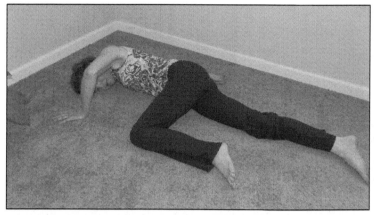

Bring your head down to look at your knee as your leg comes up.

18. After looking under your arm a few times, look above your arm the next time your left leg comes up. You'll lift your head a bit to do this. Explore this movement a few times. Make it easy and comfortable.

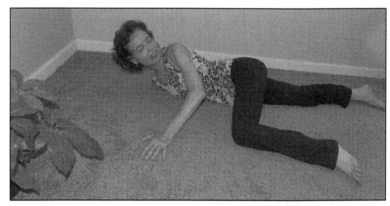

Look over your arm as you slide your leg up.

19. Go back and forth between looking under your arm and over your arm as your left leg comes up. Do that several

times, making the movements feel as easy as possible. Take a rest whenever you need to.

After several movements, take a full rest on your back. Notice the differences between your two sides. Has your ability to fully rest improved?

20. Lie on your stomach and turn your face to the right. Draw up your right leg so that it is comfortably bent. Your lower leg will still be resting on the mat. Put your left arm down by your side.

    Stand your right hand and turn your fingers outward. Find a place that allows you to push against your right hand in such a way that the force goes up into your right shoulder blade, bringing your shoulder blade closer to your spine. Put your right hand in several different places and push through your hand at each location. Try putting your hand farther away from you and then closer. Which positions make it easier to move your shoulder blade?

    Put your right hand far enough away from you that you can feel your shoulder blade slide around. Every few movements, put your hand in a different place, because every new movement will make the movement go through your body in a different path.

21. Slide your right leg down. Stand your right hand closer to your body so that you can produce power when you push through it.

    Drag up your right leg as you push against your right hand. Feel how these movements can go together. Do this several times.

22. Keep your right leg bent up. Push your right knee away from you and back toward you a few times. Feel the movement in your right hip. Make it simple and light. Feel how this movement engages the deep muscles of your core. After several movements, let your right leg go long.

23. Drag your right leg up again, but this time round your back and bring your head down to look at your knee as your leg comes up. Don't attempt to touch your head to your knee, but simply bring them toward each other. You'll be looking under your arm. Then take them apart, returning your head to the middle and letting your right leg go long. Do that movement several times.

24. After looking under your arm a few times, look above your arm the next time your right leg comes up. You'll lift your head a bit to do this. Explore this movement a few times. Make it easy and comfortable.

25. Go back and forth between looking under your arm and over your arm as your right leg comes up. Do that several times, making the movements feel as easy and novel as possible. How can you change the movement slightly each time you do it?

26. Let your right leg go long and put your forehead in the middle. Put your hands in a pushup position.

    Lift your head to look up at the wall in front of you. How easily does your head lift now? Have you learned to organize your back in a new and delightful way? When you've explored that enough, take a full rest on your back.

    Notice what has changed for you. How fully do you sense yourself now? Roll your head gently from side to side.

    Slowly roll to your side and sit up. Stand up and notice how your skeleton can effortlessly support you. Enjoy taking this feeling into your day.

Resources

Educational Products and Classes

This book is an introduction to **_Debono Moves._** To help your dog and yourself even further, we offer educational products and seminars. We plan to offer online classes soon too! Please visit **www.DebonoMoves.com/Products**.

Free Newsletter

To receive free tips to help you and your animals live happier, healthier lives, sign up for our newsletter at **http://eepurl.com/dyE2T**. You'll also be notified of Mary's events and online classes.

Workshops and Clinics

Would you like Mary to come to your town? All you need is a group of people interested in learning how to help their dogs and/or horses.

For more information, go to –
http://www.debonomoves.com/events/how-to-organize-a-workshop-or-clinic-in-your-area.

Private Sessions

Would you like to have a private session with Mary? In-person sessions (humans only) are available in Encinitas, California, USA. For more information, please visit
http://www.debonomoves.com/events/feldenkrais-method-private-sessions.

Mary also plans to offer online Skype sessions for humans and their animals so that anyone in the world can benefit from her personalized guidance. For more information, **http://www.debonomoves.com/dogs-and-cats/online-sessions-and-classes**.

Mary's husband and business partner, Gary Waskowsky, is a *Guild Certified Feldenkrais Practitioner^{cm}* who has helped people overcome physical and emotional challenges for more than 25 years. Neuro-Linguistic Programming (NLP), Emotional Freedom Technique (Meridian Tapping*)*, and *HeartMath*® biofeedback are part of the eclectic approach he offers. His work is often described as "transformational." Gary is available for online Skype sessions. His website is **www.GaryWaskowsky.com** and he can be reached at **GaryWaskowsky@gmail.com**.

Find a *Feldenkrais Method*® Practitioner

To find a *Feldenkrais* Practitioner in your area, visit **www.Feldenkrais.com**.

Locate a Holistic Veterinarian

For a list of holistic veterinarians in the United States, visit the American Holistic Veterinary Medical Association at **www.ahvma.org**.

Dog Training

Carefully interview prospective dog trainers to be certain that they use reward-based training. This is often referred to as "positive reinforcement training" or "clicker training." Always be an educated participant in your dog's training. It's generally *not* recommended that you leave your dog with a trainer.

The *Whole Dog Journal* (**www.Whole-Dog-Journal.com**), *The Bark* magazine (**www.TheBark.com**), and **www.Dogs NaturallyMagazine.com** contain insightful articles on dog training and care.

Meet the Dogs!

To view photos of the dogs featured in this book, go to **www.DebonoMoves.com/Products/Dog-Book**.

About the Author

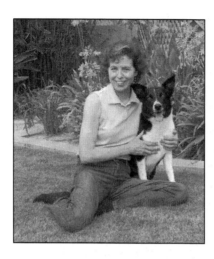

Mary Debono is a lifelong animal lover with a passion for improving the movement and well-being of animals and their people. A *Guild Certified Feldenkrais Practitioner*^{cm}, Mary began developing *Debono Moves*^{sm} (originally called the *SENSE Method)* about thirty years ago.

Mary travels internationally to teach people how to use *Debono Moves* to help their animals – and themselves – move and feel better at any age. Stories about her unique, empowering approach have appeared in numerous publications and on radio and television. In addition to her book, *Grow Young with Your Dog*, Mary and her husband, Gary Waskowsky, have developed video and audio products. Mary plans to offer online classes soon.

Mary and her husband share their lives with Ruby, a rescued Rat Terrier, and Breeze, a Quarter Horse. They make their home in San Diego County, California, USA.

Her website is **www.DebonoMoves.com**.

Made in the USA
Lexington, KY
29 November 2019